AYURVEDIC MASSAGE
FOR HEALTH AND HEALING
AYURVEDIC AND SPIRITUAL ENERGY APPROACH

AYURVEDIC MASSAGE
FOR HEALTH AND HEALING
AYURVEDIC AND SPIRITUAL ENERGY APPROACH

S.V. Govindan

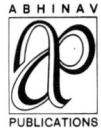

ABHINAV
PUBLICATIONS

abhinav publications

First published in India 2000
2nd edition 2006

Publishers
Shakti Malik
Abhinav Publications
E-37 Hauz Khas
New Delhi-110016 (INDIA)
Phones: 26566387, 26524658
Fax: 91-11-26857009
e-mail: shakti@nde.vsnl.net.in
website: http://www.abhinavexports.com

ISBN 81-7017-485-6

Lasertypeset by
Tara Chand Sons
Naraina, New Delhi

Printed at
D.K. Fine Art Press Pvt. Ltd.
Ashok Vihar, Delhi

Formerly published as Massage for Health and Healing

DEDICATION

We are in the world together
Not to win, not to compete
Not to conquer;
But to educate, to nurture
And to help each other,
We each the other's neighbor.
Let us celebrate
The power within us all
To forget and forgive
The faults and evils.
Let our slogan echo everywhere—
Victory of the world and peace.

—Unknown

VINOBA'S BLESSING

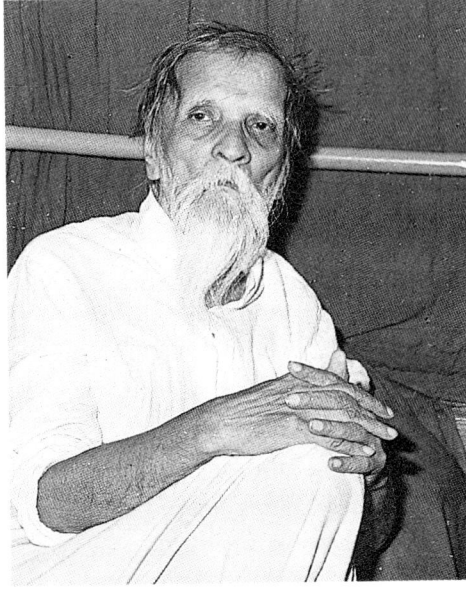

तार—फोन 2518 वर्धा

ब्रह्मविद्या मंदिर
पो० पवनार, 442111 (वर्धा)

[Handwritten Devanagari text and signature by Vinoba Bhave, dated 30-4-1981]

(Above quotation is written by Vinoba Bhave himself)

AYAM ME HASTO BHAGAWĀN	This my hand is blissful,
AYAM ME BHAGAVATTARAH	My hand is even more blissful,
AYAM ME VIŚWABHEṢAJAH	Because it contains all healing values
AYAM ŚIVĀBHIMARŚANAH	This hand's mere touch cures all
	diseases.
	—Ṛgveda

6

CONTENTS

Dedication   5
Foreword   9
Introduction   11

  I   THE BACKGROUND
    History of Massage   13
    Human Physiology   17
    Science of Marma (Vital Areas)   23

 II   WHAT IS AYURVEDIC MASSAGE?
    What is Ayurveda?   29
    Benefits and General Guidelines of Massage   35
    Cold Massage   60
    Beauty Massage for Women and Men   60
    Auto Massage   66
    Massage Movements   67
    Oils, Pastes and Essences   71
    Colors and their Effects   77
    Urine Therapy Massage   80
    Benefits of Ayurvedic Massage   83
    Ayurvedic Massages of Kerala: Pizhichil, Navarakkizhi, Dhara   85
    Doing Massage with Legs   88

 III   HEALING THROUGH MASSAGE
    Case Study Summaries   89
    Healing through Massage   90
    Ayurvedic Herbs and Food Combinations   95

 IV   SPIRITUAL ENERGY MASSAGE
    Kundalini   103
    Chakras   104
    Chakras and the Endocrine Glands   109
    Techniques of Spiritual Energy Massage   112

Appendix A: 121
    Acupressure   126
    Reflexology (Zone Therapy)

Appendix B:
  Yoga Nidra   133
  Kayakalpa   134
Charts of Marmas   137
Names and Addresses of Ayurvedic Medical Centres in Kerala 147
New Findings
 a) Shirovasti (Read before 'Doing Massage with Legs'
    on page 88)   149
 b) Infertility Problems (Read before 'General
    Injuries' on page 95)   150
 c) Meaning of So-ham (Read after the para of
    Sahasrara (Crown) Chakra on page 120)   155
 d) Photos of Yoga Asanas mentioned on page 112 157
Bibliography   159
Index   160

Page Reference of Photos

Page	Photo No.	Page	Photo No.
37	1, 11, 3	62	22, 24, 25, 23
38	2, 29, 5, 6	63	4, 28, 31
39	7, 8, 10	64	21, 32, 33, 34
40	26, 27, 45	113	38, 39, 40, 41
49	45a, 37, 30	114	42, 43, 44
50	36, 35, 9	115	46
51	12, 14, 13	152	47
52	15, 17, 16	157-158	48-55
61	20, 18, 19		

Page Reference of Figures

Page	Fig. No.	Page	Fig. No.	Page	Fig. No.
16	01	57	18	129	42
17	02	58	19	130	43
18	03	59	20, 21	150	44
19	04	68	22	151	45
22	05	69	23	151	46
24	06	70	24	152	47
25	07	88	25	153	48
26	08	93	26	154	49
43	09	103	27	154	50
45	10	109	35	154	51
46	11	115	39		
47	12	116	28 to 34		
48	13	118	36		
53	14	122	40		
54	15	124	37		
55	16	125	38		
56	17	128	41		

INTRODUCTION

Staying healthy or becoming more healthy not only requires a positive outlook but also patient, consistent maintenance of the body through massage and a healthy diet. Exercise is also advised. This book tells you how to be healthier.

This book tells you the ways and means by which you can maintain optimum health. That is what this book is all about. I have covered various topics which have a lasting and positive value for us if followed patiently with love and compassion. The benefits for both the giver and the receiver are many.

As the title suggests, this book involves an art of healing through massage. Read the book once thoroughly, treating it like a novel. Then, depending on your level of interest, read the entire book again, slowly this time, reading chapter by chapter and assimilating the contents. As you read, practice the art of massage on your spouse, parents, other relatives, or friends.

Please remember that you are entirely responsible for your health and well-being. All therapies and techniques mentioned in this book are to be adopted and followed strictly after you have consulted your personal physician.

Massage is the manipulation of the soft tissues of the body. All the theories of massage are scientific, but their application is an art developed by the individual. The masseur/masseuse should increase his/her knowledge about human anatomy and physiology, shiatsu, and acupressure in addition to carefully reading and practicing the contents of this book.

A skillful masseur/masseuse should be able to devise, in the course of his practice, better ways and means for the actual application of the various techniques. Like an artist from any discipline, a masseur/masseuse can develop his/her own style of massage but based on the basics. Hard work and regular, disciplined practice are essential. If the masseur/masseuse continues to develop his/her fingers and the sensitivity of their touch, he/she can gain dexterity that will make it possible to manipulate hidden muscles as effectively as if they were visible or on the surface of the body.

This art of massage is a God-send. The aspirant may make use of this opportunity to develop a sense of giving so that he or she is able to render a simple, yet valuable service to humanity, especially to those in need. I hope you enjoy reading this book as much as I have enjoyed writing it for you.

OM SHĀNTIH SHĀNTIH SHĀNTIH

FOREWORD TO THE SECOND EDITION

(Free rendering of the preface written for the Malayalam version)

My friend Sri S.V. Govindan is not mere a learned writer. In his early youth he was attracted by the ideals of Mahatma Gandhi and observing celibacy he proved himself as a true Satyagrahi doing constructive work for the welfare of the country. Now he is one of the old members of Vinoba's Ashram, Brahma Vidya Mandir, Paunar. He strives to achieve the ultimate and tries to serve the human beings for their physical health and spiritual peace by doing massage.

He got this art from Kelappanji. Being a regular spinner he has travelled most of the European countries and U.S.A. and Canada to propagate massage. Wherever he goes, he collects a group of friends. This experienced person is ever learning and has written some books for the benefit of others.

With his own experience he has written a small book, **Spiritual Energy Massage**. All of us know the role of acupuncture, the system of Chinese treatment. From that acupressure is developed and it is very popular everywhere. The **Spiritual Energy Massage** is based on acupressure. But the speciality is that the author has written it with his own experience. Experience is more important than definitions and commentaries.

Today the medical science goes forward breaking its boundaries for achieving the ultimate progress. Holistic vision gives enthusiasm and strength for it. So it would be better if the modern medical scientists try to understand and accept it.

The conception of yoga-chakra and the effect of Ida-Pringala and Sushumna nerves are the gifts of our ancient Indian philosophy. Now these are the subjects of great scientists for observation and study. This ancient philosophy spread to China, from China to Japan, and then it got publicity in European countries and America. With its minute study the latest system of treatment could achieve ever new dimensions. Now again it was brought to India and we accept it as their new invention. Really that is what is happening today.

Sri S.V. Govindan's **Spiritual Energy Massage** points out how far we could understand and accept such studies. I earnestly request the medical associations to read it carefully and understand. By its study, surely we will be benefited.

Arya Vaidya Sala
Kottakkal, Kerala
5-1-1995

P.K. Warrier
Managing Trustee and
Chief Physician

FOREWORD

This book on "*Massage for Health and Healing: The Ayurvedic and Spiritual Energy Approach*" is a commendable guide to a very important medical aid which reigned with dignity in the past. Though it was neglected for many years, the art of massage has recaptured its central place amongst the forms of healing, prevention of disease, and promoting health. So I consider it a privilege and an honor to write a foreword to this timely publication.

Govindanji,* a devoted social worker, is a disciple of Acharya Vinoba Bhave. He has been active in the field of Sarvodaya work for many years. The usefulness, scientific reliability, and simplicity of massage as a way to serve the masses attracted him. He wanted to help those for whom the conveniences and amenities of costly medicines were out of reach. The value of this useful technique is often overlooked, even by the enlightened. When Govindanji was initiated into this field of massage by none other than Shri K. Kelappan, a national leader from Kerala, he realized that it was one of his missions to promote this useful technique by study and propagation. By reading and observation he learned the theory and practice of massage. Encouraged by Vinobaji Bhave, Govindanji wrote his first publication in Hindi, *Mālish kā Marma*. The practicality of the book attracted many who were interested in this field. Many people read it and encouraged the author to bring out this English version of it.

Massage is the oldest of all techniques for relieving pain, shaping the organs, regenerating tissues, and correcting almost all internal malfunctions. Massage has its origin in the natural instincts of animals, handed over to the conscious man with a mandate to improve it as far as possible with his old wisdom. Despite advancements in knowledge and complex techniques, massage retains its usefulness and significance even as a method to save a person from immediate death, as in heart failure, breathlessness, and several other fatal ailments.

In all kinds of therapeutic approaches, massage alone can maintain certain links. Any method of treatment with a holistic approach cannot leave out massage. Ayurveda upholds its psychosomatic benefits. Sushruta and other texts explain it, classifying various types of massages and instructions on their manipulations and effects. In Ayurveda, the human body constitutes three functional entities, the bal-

---

*In India the addition of 'ji' at the end of a name shows respect and esteem.

ance of which maintains health; an upset in this balance increases diseases. The vital life force, energy, or prana, is regulated by the peaceful co-existence of these functional entities. This has been explained very well in this book. Massage is the most useful technique; if used in a proper way, massage can sense the specialities of the parts of the body; it can be used to correct problems. Realizing the importance of massage, all special treatments in Kerala are formulated with a holistic approach to the body and mind and have proved their efficacy in healing many complicated diseases.

This book serves not only as a guide to novice practitioners but also as a manual and refresher guide for those who are experienced ayurvedic masseurs. The contents (techniques) of this book will bring relief and better health to those who faithfully apply them in their daily lives. I am sure all those who are devoted to the study of holistic approaches will certainly appreciate this work and the author. I recommend this work to all, including research scholars, physicians, practitioners, and social and cultural workers in India and abroad.

P.K. Warrier

I THE BACKGROUND

HISTORY OF MASSAGE

The word massage, derived from Greek, signifies kneading or pressing which consists basically of palpation, rubbing and kneading. Massage is scientific manipulation of the tissues of the body.

In this modern age of the computer, nuclear and chemical warfare, a sense of each one to his own is being perpetuated either consciously or subconsciously. The feeling of oneness, the essence of being, is fast receding in our world of economic competition, in a rat race to be at the top. We tend to remember vividly the past, a past full of hatred and strife which doesn't really help in our growth and development.

Man, being a gregarious animal, cannot live as an island. Our first contact with the world is through the sense of touch. The medium, our skin, is the largest surface area as compared to the other senses. Skin has the capacity to receive varied signals and to respond to them differently. The sense of touch is the first of the five senses to become functional.

Touch can be soothing and have a healing effect. The one who touches also benefits from the experience. One of the ancient techniques of touching, healing, and curing that man has almost forgotten over the years, is the art of massage. Massage is, however, a therapeutic tool that is being revived. Many have experienced the benefits.

When I presented the manuscript of my book in Hindi to Vinobaji for his blessing, he wrote a Veda Mantra (a verse from the Rig Veda) which says, "This hand contains all healing values and this makes whole with gentle touch." Another verse of the Rig Veda says, "We, both of our hands which have ten fingers and which render the best of health, uttering mantras for health, touch you for your health."

The history of massage dates back to several centuries before our time when healers worked miracles with their hands. They worked by instinct and intuition, using techniques they developed through regular practice. Regular practice did not necessarily mean only rigorous training. It meant an unwavering discipline coupled with a certain amount of commitment on the part of the masseur/masseuse and a more essential ingredient, the feeling of oneness and harmony with the receiver.

Massage for healing had great importance in the ancient times. In those days science and technology were not very developed, but ancient Indian surgeons and physicians studied the art of massage from the famous books of Charaka, Ashtanga Hridaya, and Sushruta. Ancient warriors and soldiers had to undergo massage during their training because massage helped them to manipulate their limbs and improve their agility in general.

For thousands of years, some form of massage or other has been used to soothe and heal the sick. To the ancient Greek and Roman physicians, massage was one of the principal means of healing and relieving pain. In the fifth century B.C., Hippocrates wrote, "The physician must be experienced in many things, but assuredly in rubbing, because rubbing can bind a joint that is too loose, and can loosen a joint that is too rigid."

Pliny, a Roman naturalist, was massaged regularly to relieve his asthma. Julius Caesar was pinched all over his body to ease his neuralgia. He had intense pain along a nerve in his head because he suffered from epilepsy. During the Middle Ages, however, little was heard of massage in Europe. This was mainly due to the contempt generated for the pleasures of the flesh. It was taboo to indulge in sensual activities.

In the 19th century Per Henrik Ling, a Swedish doctor, developed the Swedish massage. He synthesized his system from his knowledge of gymnastics and physiology and from Chinese, Egyptian, Greek and Roman techniques. The first college offering massage as part of the curriculum was established in 1813 in Stockholm.

In the East, massage techniques have always been more valued for their healing applications than in the West. The scientific revolution in the West a few centuries ago has brought about an attitude that the human body is a machine which could be serviced and maintained by medical practitioners.

Today the therapeutic value of massage is again being recognized and is flourishing throughout the Western world. The countries in the East, however, continued to combine their instinctive desire of using the concept of touch with skills refined and elaborated by tradition and practice. Indians use techniques preserved in Sanskrit texts which date back to as far as 2500 B.C. These texts deal with the art of maintaining a perfect balance in the functions of the body. This system is known as Ayurveda, the science of longevity. Ayurveda is primarily concerned with the individual's habits. Following the tenets of Ayurvedic massage and diet gives freedom from physical and emotional diseases.

Ayurveda works by adjusting the intercellular fluid in the body — lymph — to create an electrical/chemical balance among organs to preserve their proper functioning. In Ayurveda, medicated oils are used for balancing DC currents in the lymph. Lymphatic massage has proven very effective in helping patients/clients to relax.

The Ayurvedic system of medicine calls the lymph system kapha (mucus carrying system). Ayurvedic massage includes pressure points which are gently massaged with organic oils such as mustard, coconut, sesame, and almond to achieve balance in the body's energy system. Ayurvedic doctors interpret kapha as being a property of lymph. Through regular massage the balance can be maintained or restored to the body's electro-chemical pathways and serve to prevent health problems. Lymphatic massage associated with marmas (vital points) has been carried forward in its most developed form into modern times by wrestlers in India.

In the West using oil to anoint a person has been known since Biblical times. Even before that Hippocrates prescribed oil anointment. Galen and Pare, and Herophilus (300 B.C.) described lymphatic vessels. In the 16th century Andreas Vesalius of Brussels and Bartolomeous Eustachius of Rome believed it to be part of a venous system. In the 17th century Olaus Rudbeck discovered that lymphatic vessels have valves that permit one-way flow of lymph as well as a separate return fluid system in the body.

The lymph system is very much taken into account in Ayurvedic massage practices. Seasonal purification is what helps man to remain healthy and strong. This purification needs to happen physically as well as mentally. The routine can start early in the morning, starting from ablution to defecating, to sweating through exercise and massage, to bathing, and finally to meditation which helps to clean the mind of negative and unwanted thoughts. These processes tend to drain out the "juices" in the body that are in excess. The body, therefore, requires oiling and lubricating to maintain its texture and moisture. The best available way for one to do it is through massage, which not only strengthens the skin but makes it soft and definitely improves its color and texture. The oil helps to reduce the erratic nature of vata and also gets rid of stiffness of the muscles.

Massaging towards the heart has a meditative quality and if oil is put into the navel, it is believed to improve the flow of prana (life force or energy) throughout the body. Massage of the head helps to calm the sense organs and also strengthen them. The shikha, the whorl at the top of the head, is the main area to be massaged. This, they say, is from where the life force or prana flows freely so as to maintain a clear consciousness.

In Indian culture, massage is a major part of our lives. Children and newborn babies are massaged until they reach a particular age. Before marriage, one undergoes the ceremonial massage. Pregnant women are massaged gently. Increase pressure gradually after delivery to help the body flush out waste material and maintain good health. Apart from the physical benefits of regular massage, the immune system of a baby is stimulated merely by the caressing touch of the mother.

In adults, however, massage should be supplemented by more regular exercise

BONES

Front View   Back View

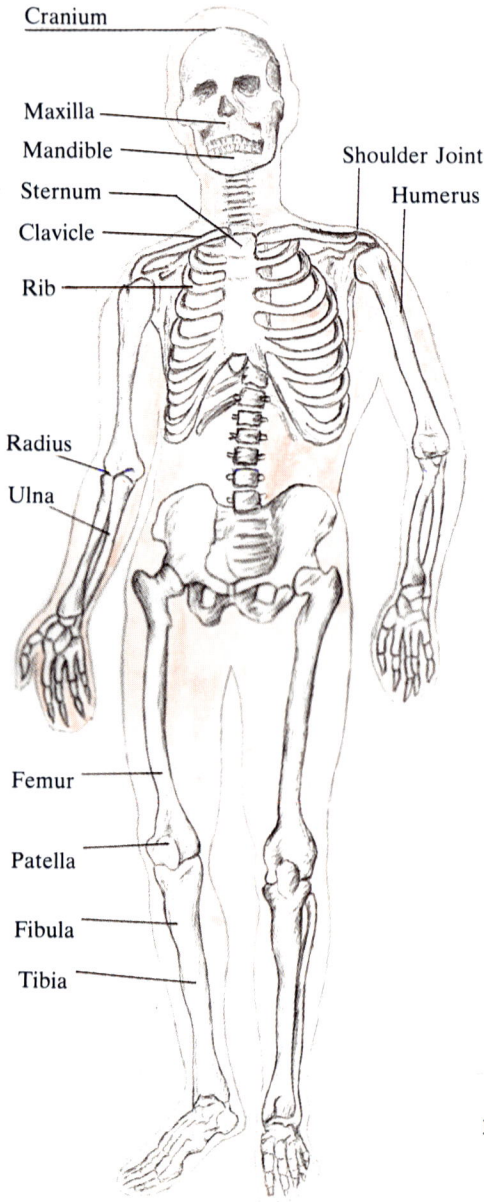
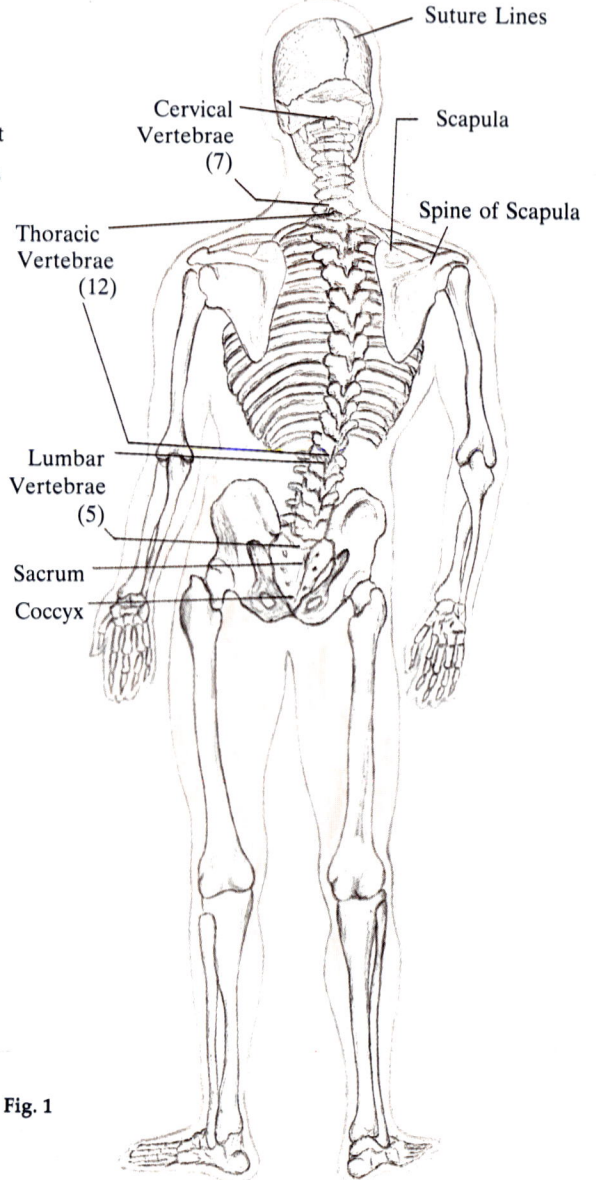

Cranium

Maxilla

Mandible

Sternum   Shoulder Joint

Clavicle   Humerus

Rib

Radius

Ulna

Femur

Patella

Fibula

Tibia

Suture Lines

Cervical
Vertebrae   Scapula
(7)

Thoracic   Spine of Scapula
Vertebrae
(12)

Lumbar
Vertebrae
(5)

Sacrum

Coccyx

Fig. 1

and perfect control over the diet. The maintaining of a good physique is just as important as acquiring it. Active exercise (massage being passive) helps in gearing up various systems in the body, to function at an optimum level, so that, with the free flow of the life force, all diseases and ailments can be kept at bay.

HUMAN PHYSIOLOGY

A general knowledge of the human anatomy, especially for someone who is training to be a masseur or masseuse, is very important and necessary. Massage activates the spine, muscles, skin, blood vessels, nerves, joints and bones. Nature has

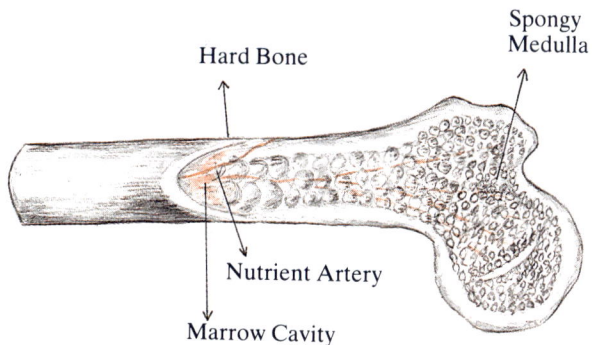

Spongy Medulla

Hard Bone

Nutrient Artery

Marrow Cavity

THE KNEE JOINT
The knee is the body's largest joint. It is a hinge joint that can move in one plane only, like the hinge of a door.

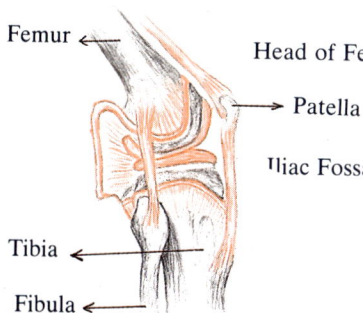

THE HIP JOINT
Like all ball-and-socket joints, the hip has a round head that fits into a cupped socket, allowing movement in any direction.

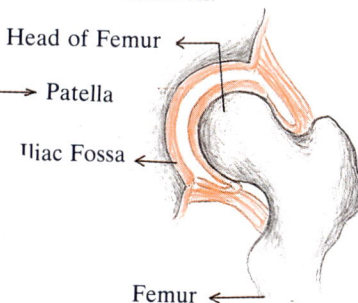

Femur

Head of Femur

Patella

Iliac Fossa

Tibia

Fibula

Femur

Fig. 2

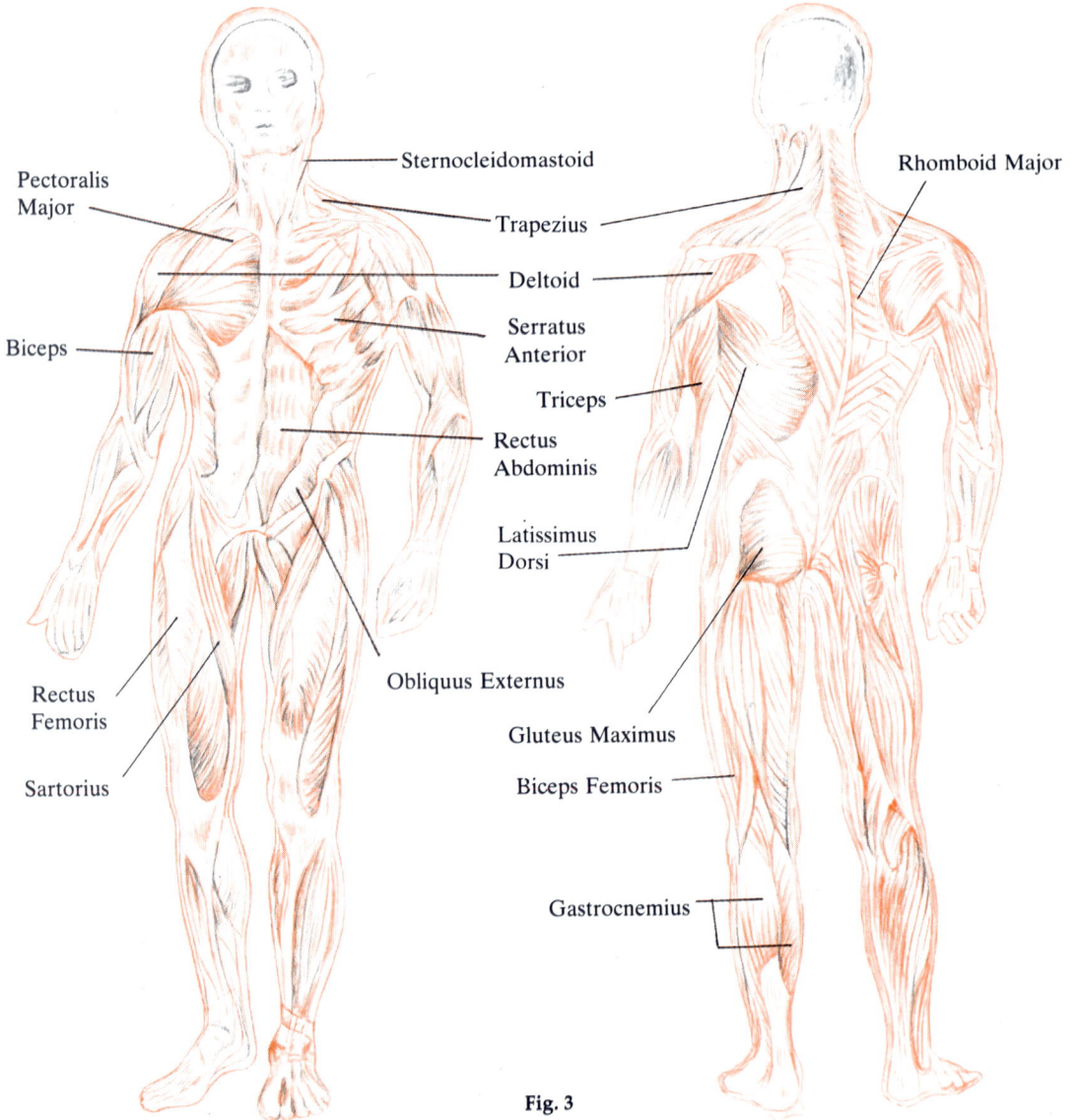

MUSCLES

Front View   Back View

Pectoralis
Major

Sternocleidomastoid   Rhomboid Major

Trapezius

Deltoid

Biceps

Serratus
Anterior

Triceps

Rectus
Abdominis

Latissimus
Dorsi

Obliquus Externus

Rectus
Femoris

Gluteus Maximus

Sartorius

Biceps Femoris

Gastrocnemius

Fig. 3

Superficial Muscles   Deep Muscles   Superficial Muscles   Deep Muscles

NERVOUS SYSTEM

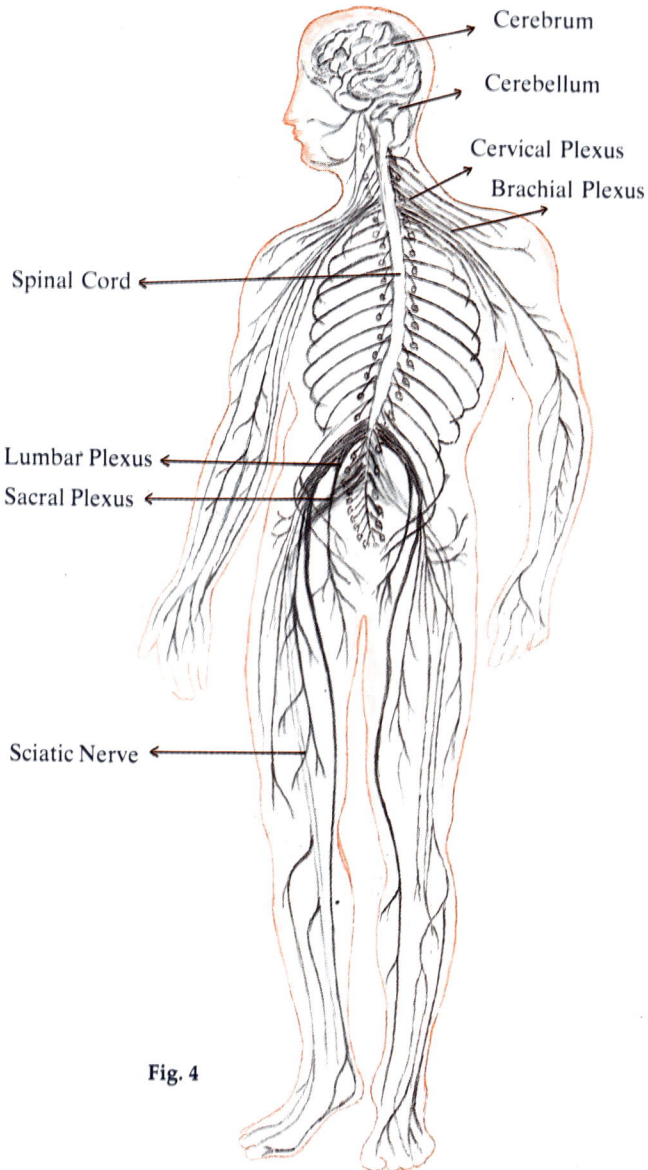

Cerebrum

Cerebellum

Cervical Plexus

Brachial Plexus

Spinal Cord

Lumbar Plexus

Sacral Plexus

Sciatic Nerve

Fig. 4

provided every human being with an in-built mechanism to repair damaged parts and to maintain good health. A masseur's/masseuse's understanding of the anatomy will enable him/her to tackle root causes of various problems. Studying human anatomy and physiology, starting from the architecture of bones and muscles, the nervous system, and skin, will help you understand the energy inherent in the human body.

Bones. All bones are moist and active, and require nourishment. They have a hard outer covering and a porous inner portion called the bone marrow. Bone marrow serves as an important mineral reserve and also helps to produce red blood cells. Bones make up the skeleton, the flexible framework of the body (Figure 1). They not only support the body and protect the most delicate organs, but also make movement possible. They act as levers at the joints, the points of connection between them.

Joints. The meeting point of two or more bones is called a joint (Figure 2). In structure and function, joints vary enormously. The body has many kinds of joints, strong mobile joints in the limbs, immobile ones that link the bones of the skull, hinge joints in the knees, elbows, and ankles, and ball and socket joints in the hips and shoulders. The ends of the bones in free moving joints are covered with cartilage and linked by a smooth tissue called the synovial membrane. This secretes a synovial fluid which lubricates the joints. Production of the synovial fluid is stimulated by massage.

Muscles. Muscles are overlapping bundles of fibers or cells, supplied with blood, lymph and nerves. Tendons at the ends of muscles attach to the bones. Muscles enable us to move and give shape to our bodies. They also help us to breathe, digest food, and circulate blood.

Muscles are either voluntary or involuntary. Skeletal muscles (Figure 3) are attached to a bone on either side of the joint. Most muscles work in pairs, one moving the joint in one direction and the other in the opposite direction. The skeletal muscles are placed symmetrically on either side of the body. Massage helps to dispel the hard knots caused by muscular spasms due to chronic tension, emotional or physical stress or trauma.

Circulation. The circulatory system transports blood throughout the body. It transports oxygen and other nutrients to the cells, removes waste products, and destroys invading bacteria with the help of the white blood corpuscles. The main organ involved with the circulation of blood is the heart, which transports about ten and a half pints of blood per minute when the body is at rest and up to 42 pints during strenuous exercise. An average adult human body contains 12 pints of blood. The purified oxygenated blood is pumped out by the heart and this travels through the arteries of the body to tiny blood vessels called capillaries, where the oxygen and nutrients are exchanged for carbon dioxide and other waste products. Waste laden blood is brought back to the heart through veins; the heart in turn sends the blood to the lungs for purification. The air we breathe oxygenates the impure blood. Veins are generally closer to the surface than the arteries. Massage aids circulation by assisting venous flow to the heart which helps to eliminate waste, lower pressure, and increase oxygen in the tissues.

Heart. Nature's own pumping device in the human body is the heart which pumps and circulates bright red oxygenated blood that comes through the pulmonary veins to the left auricle and ventricle of the heart, from the lungs and in turn from the heart through the aorta, through the arteries to the different parts of the body. The impure deoxygenated blood is brought back to the right auricle and ventricle of the heart and then through the pulmonary arteries to the lungs for recycling.

The heart of an adult beats 72 times per minute. A baby up to 6 months has 140 to 115 beats per minute; a child up to 4 years has 120 to 105 beats per minute. A child up to 6 years has 115 to 90 beats per minute, while a 10 year old has between 90 to 80. A 15 year old has 85 to 75 beats per minute. In old age the pulse rate increases. At any age a person's pulse rate may increase due to fever, fear, anxiety, or anger. Most people breathe 18 times per minute with breath to heart ratio of 1 : 4.

Lymphatic system. The lymphatic system helps to maintain the correct fluid balance in the tissues and blood to defend the body against diseases and to remove waste products. It has an intricate filtering system made up of tiny lymph vessels which circulate lymph, a milky fluid, through the body. The movement of the lymph is affected by massage which helps to propel the fluid through the body. In the course of circulation, lymph vessels carry excess fluid and bacteria from the tissues that are filtered out by lymph nodes or glands in the neck, armpits, groin, and knees as well as in certain other parts of the torso. Massage stimulates the lymphatic flow and helps in the removal of lactic acid and other waste material generated in the body due to excessive exercise.

Nervous system. The nervous system receives inputs from internal as well as external stimuli, then it decodes and stores them in the brain, and generates certain behavior in response (Figure 4). The central nervous system is comprised of the brain and the spinal cord which form a two-way communication channel linked to all other parts of the body. The spinal and cranial nerves are voluntary. Involuntary nerves are responsible for functions such as digestion and respiration. Sensory nerves convey impulses from receptors in the sense organs to the spinal cord and the brain. Motor nerves convey information and instruction from the brain to the organs and tissues through the spinal cord. The nervous system reacts to the environment appropriately and regulates the activities of the other body systems by relaxing and toning the nerves. Massage improves the functioning and condition of all the organs of the body.

NERVE ZONES

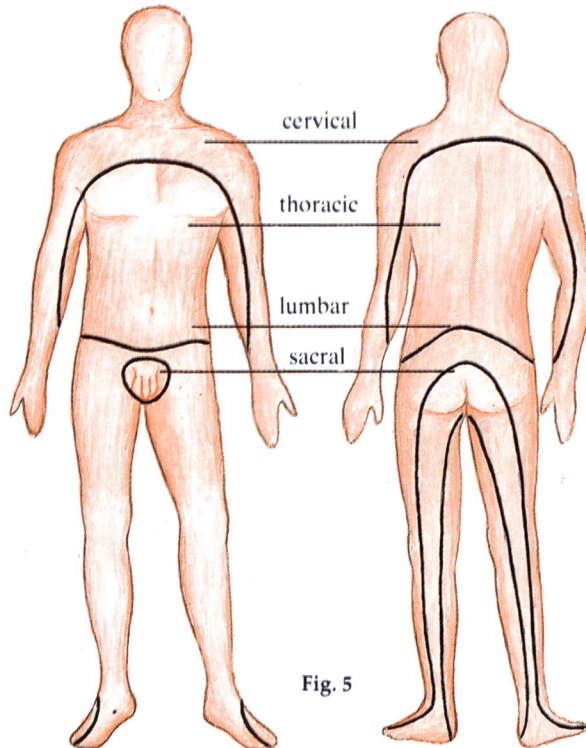

cervical

thoracic

lumbar

sacral

Fig. 5

Spinal nerves branch out from the spinal cord in pairs to serve different parts of the body. The neck and arms are supplied by nerves from the cervical area, the rib cage and abdomen by nerves from the thoracic area, the lower back, hip and front of the legs by nerves from the lumbar area, and the base of the legs by nerves from the sacral area (Figure 5). Knowledge of the areas of the body, serviced by the various spinal nerves, is essential and important while massaging the body for treatment. For example, to eliminate sciatic pain while massaging, the masseur/ masseuse should concentrate on the sacral area of the spine in addition to along the back of the legs. Aching hip joints may be relieved by massaging the lumbar area as well as the aching joint.

Skin. The skin, the organ of touch, is the largest organ of the body. It provides strong waterproof protection for the underlying parts. Skin also helps to eliminate waste material from the body and to regulate temperature. The abundant supply of nerve endings helps to absorb information from the environment. The receptor cells are very sensitive to light, touch, pain, heat, and cold. Other receptor cells are situated in the skin which eliminates waste through perspiration. The sebaceous glands secrete an oily substance which aids in keeping the skin supple and moist and protected from bacteria.

SCIENCE OF MARMA (VITAL AREAS)

The word marma (vital area) is described in the Hindu scripture *Atharva Veda*. During the Vedic period knowledge of the vital areas of the human body became part of military science. This knowledge was applied in war, medicine, and surgery. Science of Marma was developed by the physicians and surgeons of Vedic period to prevent death and treat people suffering from trauma.

The vital areas are more prone to complications caused by injury than other parts of the body. With the advancement and progress of modern surgery and medicine, it has become an essential part of the duty of an ayurvedic anatomist to explore the non-clinical and clinical value of these vital areas in the human body, as discussed by ancient physicians and surgeons. A marma, defined as an anatomical area where flesh, veins, arteries, tendons, bones and joints meet to form the seats of life, has secret and significant valves at these junctions. The anatomical areas where structures pulsate and where pain exists can be labelled marmas.

Warriors usually targeted important marmas on the bodies of the enemy to inflict maximum damage. Physicians and surgeons used the same knowledge to heal these wounds. Sushruta classified these marmas on the basis of their location in the body, dimension, and the effect of injuries. In all he classified 107 marmas.

Marmas are classified into three sections: structural, regional, and prognostic. The marmas are classified according to their location in the body and the effect of any kind of impact or injury to the particular marma in question.

Structural Marmas. This classification, according to human physiology, includes:

Muscles — 11
Blood vessels (veins and arteries) — 41
Ligaments (tendons) — 27
Bones — 8
Vulnerable areas — 20

Regional Marmas. In the regional classification, the marmas are divided according to the organs and sections of the body:

Upper limbs — 22
Lower limbs — 22
Abdomen and thorax — 12
Back of the trunk — 14
Head and neck — 37 (see Figures 6-8)

MARMAS I

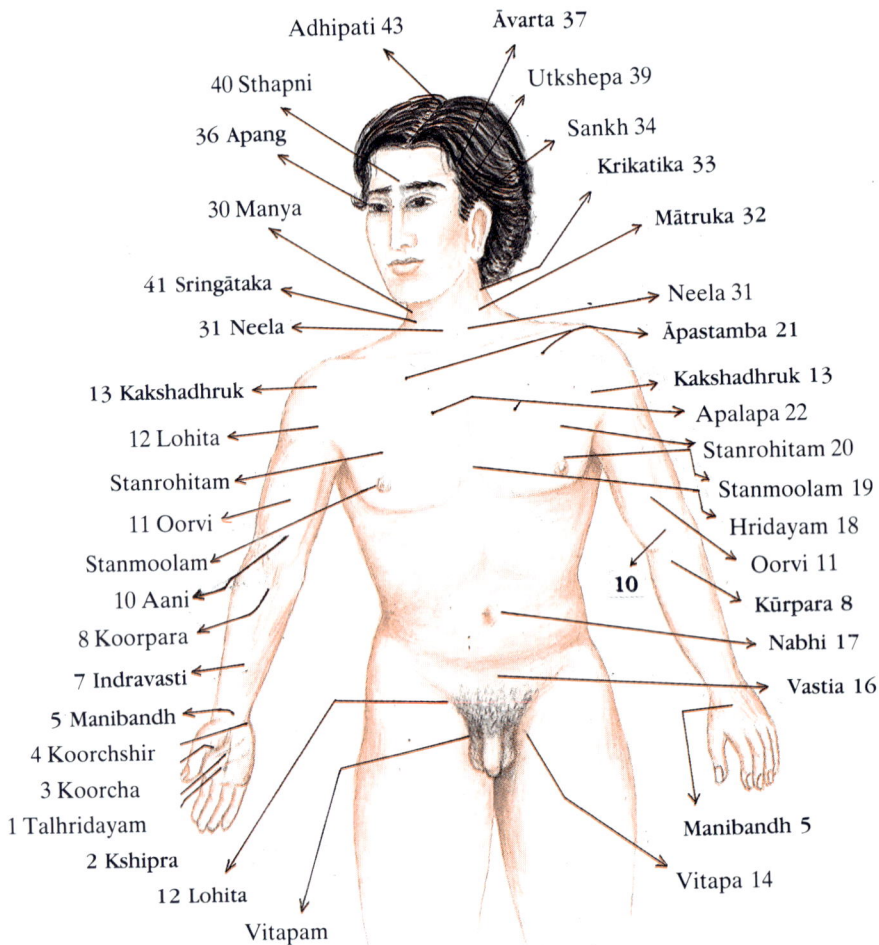

Adhipati 43   Āvarta 37

40 Sthapni   Utkshepa 39

36 Apang   Sankh 34

                                Krikatika 33

30 Manya   Mātruka 32

41 Sringātaka   Neela 31

31 Neela   Āpastamba 21

13 Kakshadhruk   Kakshadhruk 13

12 Lohita   Apalapa 22

Stanrohitam   Stanrohitam 20

11 Oorvi   Stanmoolam 19

Stanmoolam   Hridayam 18

10 Aani   Oorvi 11

8 Koorpara   10   Kūrpara 8

7 Indravasti   Nabhi 17

5 Manibandh   Vastia 16

4 Koorchshir

3 Koorcha

1 Talhridayam

2 Kshipra   Manibandh 5

12 Lohita   Vitapa 14

Vitapam

Fig. 6

MARMAS II

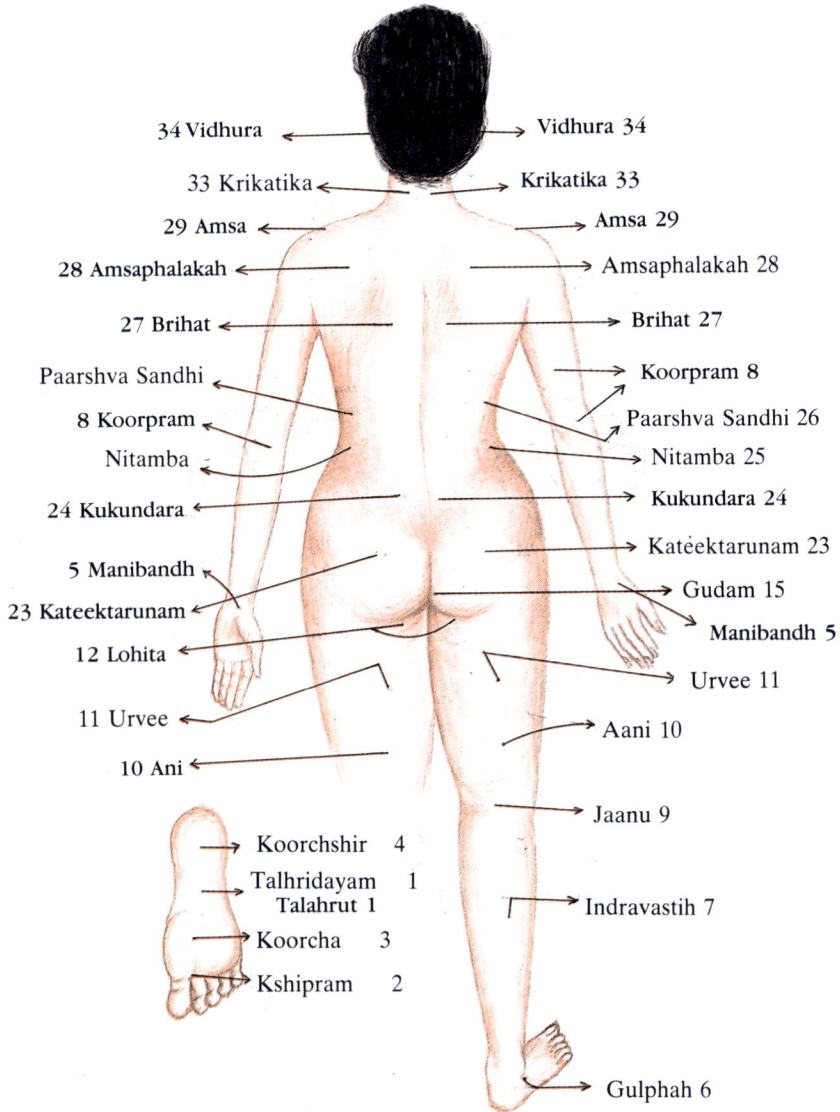

34 Vidhura   Vidhura 34

33 Krikatika   Krikatika 33

29 Amsa   Amsa 29

28 Amsaphalakah   Amsaphalakah 28

27 Brihat   Brihat 27

Paarshva Sandhi   Koorpram 8

8 Koorpram   Paarshva Sandhi 26

Nitamba   Nitamba 25

24 Kukundara   Kukundara 24

5 Manibandh   Kateektarunam 23

23 Kateektarunam   Gudam 15

12 Lohita   Manibandh 5

11 Urvee   Urvee 11

10 Ani   Aani 10

Koorchshir   4   Jaanu 9

Talhridayam   1
Talahrut 1   Indravastih 7

Koorcha   3

Kshipram   2

Gulphah 6

Fig. 7

MARMAS III

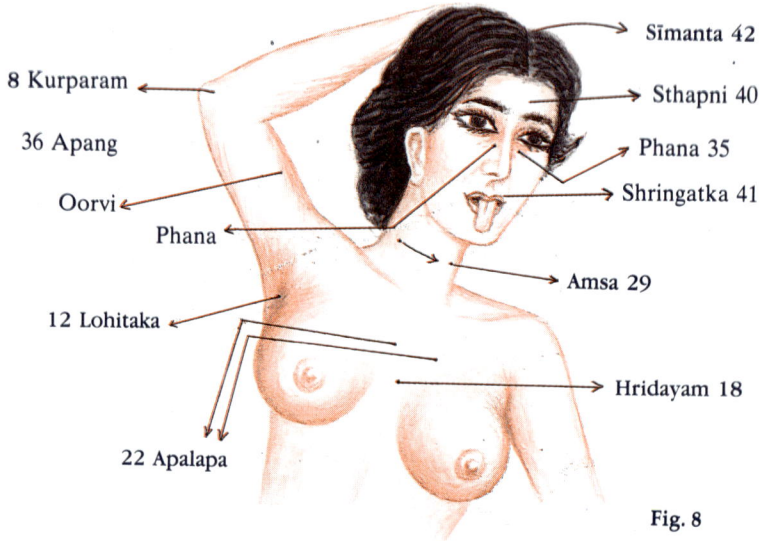

Fig. 8

Prognostic Marmas. Any symptom from which one can diagnose diseases is called prognosis. The marmas in this category are classified according to the effects of injuries on these marmas:

Slow death — 33
Disability — 44
Pain — 8

For the marmas mentioned below, a general body massage, consisting mainly of rubbing, is sufficient. Care must be taken to use the best massage techniques because applying too much pressure can cause injury.

Muscle Marma. One of the characteristics of the living organism is its capability to react appropriately to changes around it due to electrical, chemical, pathogenic, or mechanical stimuli. The human being can make the most appropriate, effective responses when the system is in excellent physical and mental condition. At the site of the mechanical response, the action gets expelled out. The muscles also prossess the power which is capable of initiating contraction. The association of muscles with bones and their innervation by ligaments (tendons) or nerves and blood vessels (veins and arteries) transforms them into the most effective system, capable of protecting the body from external trauma or injuries.

Vishalyaghna Marma. Some marmas in the body, like the Sthapani marma, are situated in between the eyes. If an arrow strikes a person at this marma, he will not die suddenly because contact is maintained with the marma by the arrow. The moment the arrow is removed, the contact is lost and the person will die. These marmas are 3 in number. Sudden death marmas number 19.

Blood Vessel Marma. Blood vessels, known by the names of veins and arteries, are distributed throughout the body as a series of tubes ranging from small to large. These form a network which is subdivided into minute vessels. If any of these blood vessels is torn, punctured, or injured at a vital site or area, the nutrition to that vital part is restricted, ultimately leading to loss of function, pain, and sometimes even death.

Bone Marma. From the orthopedic point of view, bone is an important part of the anatomy. Injuries and diseases of bones are considered under the subject of Orthopedic Traumatology. The extent of injury to a bone depends upon the mechanical or physical force of impact.

Ligament Marma/Tendon Marma. The purpose of ligaments is to prevent abnormal movements at a joint though some of the tendons are better protected by muscles than others. For example, the collateral tendons of the knee and inferior tibiofibular tendons are poorly protected. Injury or trauma to such tendons can cause permanent damage or lead to a sprain due to the rupture of a ligament.

Joint Marma. All movements that include locomotion are accomplished by the bending or straightening of the limbs (arm, forearm, hands, thighs, legs and feet), or of the trunk itself. Therefore, all vertebrates possess joints. Joint injuries are commonly classified as dislocation, sub-laxation, and sprains. The most common cause of these is a trauma or injury.

Though the practical application of the knowledge of body marmas disappeared, it persists in Kerala among the practitioners of the martial art known as Kalarippayattu. According to Kalarippayattu, injury to a marma blocks or cuts the associated nadi (tendon or pulse) at the point, interrupting both the flow of life force and the flow of life force's waste product vata. Immediate first aid for such an injury is firm stroking and slapping to the similar marma on the opposite side of the body to get the life force moving again, to get the victim out of danger. Such a counterapplication must be given within a short time for it to work. This action must be followed by Ayurvedic treatment of the injury. The life force's movements through as well as concentration in marmas is controlled by the lunar day. This doctrine of marmas is strikingly similar to that of Indian sexology which details specific areas of a woman that are awake to erotic excitement on particular lunar days because of the movement of the life forces therein.

Some marmas are not classified like the above-mentioned marmas. In olden times, when there was no anesthesia or chloroform for surgery, expert Ayurvedic physician used to press certain points on the patient's body by which the patient would become unconscious. After having administered the necessary treatment, he would press another set of points to bring the patient back to consciousness. A similar process was used for local anesthesia also.

The study of Marmas and keeping them in mind would be sometimes very necessary to the masseur/masseuse. Patients who have injury on such vital areas, by regular massage get relief and they may overcome their disabilities. Hence general knowledge of Marmas would be useful.

Those who want to know more about Marmas they can refer to the details of Marmas with figures in 'Charts of Marmas'.

I have divided the 107 marmas in the regional format with the appropriate figure so that it becomes easy for the masseur to locate the required marma. In the normal condition all areas of marmas can be massaged without more pressure.

II WHAT IS AYURVEDIC MASSAGE?

WHAT IS AYURVEDA?

Ancient History

Ayurveda means "the knowledge of life" or "the course of life". This compound word consists of ayuh which means life and veda which means knowledge. Hinduism is based on ancient texts called the vedas. The vedas are texts of hymns and collections of experiences of the sages and other wise men of yore. The four main branches of the vedas are: the Rig Veda, consisting mainly of hymns; the Yajur Veda, consisting of procedures for various sacrifices; the Sama Veda, with Rig Vedic hymns set to tune, and the Atharva Veda, dealing with the healing arts.

Ayurveda is an offshoot or an accessory of the Atharva Veda which deals with the curative aspect or the white magic section of the Veda. Ayurveda, essentially being the science of life, considers the treatment of diseases as an important branch, since health has to be restored and maintained. However, Atharva Veda makes references to other Vedas about treatment. Ayurveda has incorporated the use of natural substances such as herbs, roots, leaves, and stems, thus bringing forth this science of medicine. These combinations of herbs and other ingredients were used not only for curative purposes but also for the prevention of diseases as well as the maintenance of optimum health.

Apart from the Atharva Veda, the Rig Veda is also said to contain many verses and mantras (similar to hymns) which denote the importance of the maintenance of health and hygiene in a human being. According to Indian mythology, Ayurveda was first perceived, not composed. Some historical sources say that Daksha Prajapati taught this science to the Ashwinikumars, who were considered to be celestial physicians. Other texts vary in their views. According to Sushruta Samhita, Lord Dhanwantari learned the art from Lord Indra, who is believed to be the king of the Gods. Whereas the Charaka Samhita believes that Bharadwaj and Atreya learned it from Indra. The Brahma Vaivarta Purana says that Bhaskara composed the Ayurveda on the advice of Daksha Prajapati.

Man is believed to go through four stages of life. The first is the study period, followed by work and raising a family. The third is retirement from the family, with more concentration on social work, and fourth and finally, renunciation. Vedanta, an era that started after the Vedic era, preached these four stages of a man's life. Thus many began to adopt renunciation as a way of life. Therefore the new Ayurvedic tradition that developed put stress on passing medical knowledge down from renunciative gurus to renunciative disciples. This knowledge was not for commercial purposes like it was used earlier, but was meant for their own use and free treatment of anyone who might come to them.

In the post-Vedic period, Ayurvedic medical practitioners developed eight specialized branches:

Internal Medicine
General Surgery
Treatment of diseases of the Head and Neck
Pediatrics
Toxicology
Science of Aphrodisiacs
Science of Rejuvenation
Psychiatry (including the treatment of diseases caused by evil spirits)

Charaka and Sushruta were the earliest medical practitioners. The medical manuals that these two great men produced are still followed as texts by those who are training in the field of Ayurvedic medicine. In those days, the *Charaka Samhita* and the *Sushruta Samhita* were written to guide and even train doctors to treat the people from the king to captains of industry. Charaka was more of physician and excelled in internal medicine, while Sushruta was a surgeon and believed that surgery was the best form of treatment, as it produced immediate results. Ayurveda is much more than a medical system. It is really a state of mind. It is a universal art of healing, which has survived even some of the strongest social revolutions and cultural changes.

The most available Ayurvedic classics (writings) are *Charaka Samhita* and *Sushruta Samhita* written during the 7th century B.C. During the medieval period rasa sastra (chemistry) became an important part of Ayurveda. During foreign invasions and internal fights, many original Ayurvedic works were destroyed.

Orientalists, especially in Europe, evinced interest in Ayurveda and had made a special study. They studied the Tridosha theory of Indian medicine correlating it with the moral theory of Arabs and Greeks. Tridosha theory explains physiology of the human body and provides the foundation of Ayurvedic medicine on which prevention and healing of all diseases are firmly based—for the benefit of mankind. The Tridoshas of the Ayurvedic system have very little in common with the theory of humors in the West.

Tridoshas

Ayurveda is based on the three doshas (dosha is an error, a fault which is against the cosmic rhythm leading to disharmony), which are invisible forces of nature. They are manifested in living beings as different characteristics. The three doshas are vata, pitta, and kapha. Vata comes from air and ether; pitta (bile) comes from fire and water, and kapha (phlegm or mucus) from earth and water. These three doshas do not belong on the physical plane though they help to keep the balance of the body. Balance is attained by the continuous flow of these three doshas out of the body. They are manifested physically and excreted.

Excess kapha or phlegm is removed from the body through urine. Sweating helps to remove excess pitta (bile) from the system, and excess vata (wind) is removed through the feces. Continuous and balanced elimination of these three doshas helps to maintain healthy levels of vata, pitta, and kapha within the body. An imbalance in any one of the three leads to disease. All three doshas are interrelated and it is important to know that without them, our daily lives would be difficult.

Vata is kinetic energy (all motion of body and mind), hence it is capable of conducting both motor and sensory functions of the body. The knowledge of vata is situated in the head, therefore concluding that the seat of vata is the central nervous system (especially below the hip), which is rich in fluids and has nerve impulses. Vata travels through nerve fibers and is maintained by the nerve fibers themselves. The general functions of vata include motor functions, synthesis of motor and sensory functions, biochemical functions, division and differentiation of cells and functions related to emotions. Vata is predominant in old age.

Pitta is responsible for transformation and mutation in the body. Pitta means to burn, to generate and enable a person to follow a proper routine. The function of pitta is performed by substances like various digestive enzymes, vitamins, and hormones which generate heat and help in the digestion of food. Pitta promotes digestion, power of vision, production of normal body heat, and maintenance of the normal complexion of the body. Hence the seat of pitta is in the stomach. Pitta is also responsible for some of mental functions such as intelligence, memory. It gives courage, cheerfulness, and lucidity of the mind. This dosha is predominant in a person's youth.

Kapha is formed by the predominance of water and earth; it produces the stabilizing influence in the human being. The general functions of kapha are viscidity, binding of joints, and stability. It promotes bulk, contributes to sexual potency and the capacity to reproduce, and strength and resistance to diseases and decay. Kapha is seated in the chest, head (including the nose and neck), joints, and upper part of the stomach. This dosha is predominant in a person's childhood.

How a human being feels inside physically depends on the working of the doshas. At the emotional level also, the doshas tend to influence the personality of the person. So it is to your advantage to change your constitution to the appropriate one, depending on your strengths and weaknesses, so that you can definitely and truly lead a happy and contented life. This would mean both health and wealth wise.

Ayurveda teaches that diseases normally spread during a change in the season. These changes affect what takes place inside the system; each person needs the capacity to adapt to them. If a person undergoes regular purification cycles, at the junction of two seasons, then the chances of contracting diseases are reduced. Purification cycles mean changing food habits, again pertaining to the doshas. Vata is cold, clear, light, subtle, and mobile. Pitta is slightly oily, intense, sour, light, hot, and mobile. Kapha is cold, heavy, oily, stable, soft, and smooth. Going by these properties, appropriate foods can be taken so as to maintain the balance. Pitta and vata are lighter when compared to kapha, which is heavy. Kapha and vata are cold while pitta is hot. Pitta and kapha are oily and moist while vata is dry. Spicy food increases pitta, dry food increases vata and anything heavy increases kapha. For example, puffed rice has vata properties, mustard oil has pitta properties, and yogurt has kapha properties.

The onset of diseases does not depend upon food habits alone. It can involve various activities that people indulge in during the course of a day in their lives. Every human being must take precautions to control the predominant dosha in his/her system to maintain balance all round the year. Generally speaking one needs to control vata during early winter, kapha during late winter and spring, and pitta during the summer.

The kind of food that you eat does play a very important role in your health and well-being. A section in this book focuses on Ayurvedic herbs, their properties, the advantages and disadvantages of their consumption, and characteristics, an ideal diet as well as a routine for an aspirant of good health to follow.

Ayurveda is not just a system of medicine based on humoral theory of disease. Its importance springs from the fact that it reflects the law of nature inherent in life. Ayurveda has a definite edge in the rules of personal conduct for longevity because it gives detailed instructions about personal hygiene, sleep during the day, diet, and so on, that impinges on a healthy life.

Ayurveda is holistic and is centered on the person rather than the disease. It points out that the mind, soul, and body are like a tripod, each leg is essential.

The Ayurvedic emphasis on the wholeness of the person is reflected in the comprehensiveness of the diagnostic examination. The physician collates and compares the information of the different orders of being, taking into account the three types of land — arid, marshy, and ordinary; three types of temperament with

16 sub-types, three bases of physical differentiation with 20 sub-types and three ages of human being (childhood, youth, many people would add middle age, and old age). All this shows the emphasis of Ayurveda. Ayurveda is essentially a science of healing which concentrated on the techniques of a healthy, normal life.

Of the three humors (vata, pitta, kapha), vata (wind) occupies the most prominent position. Food moves into the stomach and blood circulates by the power of prāna vāyu. The apāna is the region of the anus and acts downward to expel feces, urine, semen or ova, and fetuses. The samāna, located in the navel, helps in the digestion of food and transforms it into blood, semen, and urine. When any of the three humors increases disproportionately in relation to the others, the healthy balance is lost and disease may result. Any loss of dynamic balance may be due to excessive (1) objects of the senses, (2) action (mind, body, speech), and (3) time (season).

One cardinal rule of Ayurveda is that medicine cannot be prescribed unless the physician has taken into account the patient's constitution, because a drug which helps one type of constitution may not help another person with a different constitution.

Those who practice Ayurveda believe that illness results from the disturbance of the equilibrium that must remain among the three humors. Any loss of that balance makes a person susceptible to manifold disorders.

Diagnosis. According to Ayurveda, health is a state of balance among the three humors (doshas) and also body, mind, and soul should be in a natural state. So the physician emphasizes a regimen of diet with the use of appropriate drugs. The age of the patient, the climate in which he lives, his cultural and social surroundings, and his bodily constitution need to be taken into account before offering a prognosis. Touch, inspection, and interrogation are the main tools of diagnosis. In Ayurveda the diagnosis is more subjective than objective. But the comprehensiveness of the examination offsets any deficiencies because of the subjectivity of the diagnosis.

Ayurvedic practitioners never deny the existence of germs, but they do not give priority to the aetiology of physical disorders. If a person has a mucus constitution he would more easily fall prey to infection of the throat, bronchial tubes, and lungs than another in whom the humor is not vitiated. Experiments conducted in the United States have proved that even the introduction of cancerous cells into healthy bodies will not produce cancer in all cases. That shows that germs are not the only reason.

The entire body of the patient is palpitated to find out the normal and abnormal condition, whether a particular organ or the entire system is cold or hot, moist or dry, light or heavy, sensitive or insensitive, rough or smooth, rigid or loose, depressed or elevated.

The three humors when increased manifest their characteristic symptoms in proportion to the intensity of their morbidity. When decreased they cease to manifest their characteristic qualities. When normal they perform the normal functions of the body. Attention also needs to be paid to the condition of various channels because blockade of these channels gives rise to disease. Blockage of the bile ducts results in jaundice. Scanty passage of the urine can cause a rise to an abnormal proportion of uric acid in the blood.

The normal function of the vāta (wind) sustains the body; it is the originator of every kind of action of the body. As the wind controls the direction of clouds, vāta controls the function of bile and mucus.

The five vayus are listed:

(1) Prāna is responsible for breathing, swallowing food, functioning of the heart, and all parts of the body directly connected with it.

(2) Udāna is responsible for the production of various sounds and speech, action and efforts to keep up the strength of the body, mind, memory, and intellect.

(3) Samāna controls the flow of the nourishment of the body. It helps digestion. It separates the essences for the nourishment of the body and sends the wastes to the large intestine.

(4) Apāna holds the feces, urine, mucus, and semen or ovum up to a normal period and expels them through the various orifices of the body. It is one of the most important vayus as it keeps the body healthy.

(5) Vyāna flows in the whole body and carries food juice and blood throughout the body. It helps secretions of perspiration and controls the opening and closing of the eyelids and other movements of the body.

Pitta

(1) Pāchaka pitta is responsible for digestion of food. It divides the food juice into fine and waste parts, and then helps the other four pittas to function normally.

(2) Ranjaka pitta gives color to the food juice when it goes from the stomach to the liver.

(3) Sādhaka, the finest of all, helps the normal functioning of the intellect and memory.

(4) Ālochaka is responsible for the maintenance of normal vision of the eyes.

(5) Bhrajaka is in the skin and is responsible for the normal color of the skin.

Mucus

(1) Kledaka is responsible for moistening the food in the stomach, nourishes the other mucus by its special humid properties.

(2) Avalambaka is at the thorax and protects the heart from excessive heat and gives a special power to the heart.

(3) Bodhaka moistens any substance contacted with the tongue and helps to know the taste. It is at the root of the tongue to the throat. It increases appetite.

(4) Tarpaka cools the organs of the senses of sight and hearing.

(5) Shleshaka is at the joints of the body and maintains them in good order, firm but also free to move.

Six factors for digestion
1. Pāchaka pitta or digestive fire
2. Samāna vayu
3. Moisture
4. Kledaka mucus
5. Time
6. Proper combination of the first five

Six types of taste (see section on food)

Sweet, sour, salty, pungent, bitter, astringent. The food is subject to the action of bodhaka and kledaka mucus in the mouth and upper part of the stomach. Sweet digestive action is followed by the action of bile when the digestive fire dries up the waste product which goes into the large intestine. Mucus is the by-product of rasa dhatu (humor of the body), bile, urine, sweat, facial fat, secretion of the genitalia, secretions of various orifices of the body like ears, eyes, nose, mouth. Doshas (humors) are defects, the imbalance among which gives rise to diseases.

BENEFITS AND GENERAL GUIDELINES OF MASSAGE

Massage is necessary for every creature, animal or human. A unique factor of nature is that even grass, plants and trees get massaged every time the wind blows through them. Everybody, either knowingly or unknowingly, definitely practices massage. In order to keep one's health, awareness, and longevity, massage is very essential. With massage, the physical appearance of the body is enhanced to a very great extent. The complexion and quality of the skin undergoes a transformation. Massage helps to cure various ailments ranging from paralysis to insomnia. Daily massage strengthens the muscles and restores strength and vitality. Massage is very essential for being more youthful and for minimizing the effects of old age, as are exercises and sports.

Haphazard eating, drinking and sleeping habits often cause more harm than good to this wonderful gift of God, the human body. Even if a person has misused and abused Nature's gift for a long time, massage can help us to restore the body to its normal condition of health, vitality, youth, stamina, and awareness. Massage benefits all parts of the human body. It aids in digestion, absorption and assimilation. It stimulates the nutrition of the body by the circulation of fresh blood and causing an interchange of fluids within the tissues. It also removes inflammation and swelling and disperses congestion. In cases of orthopedic ailments masseur/masseuse gives good results.

General Benefits. Massage has an overall effect on the immune system of the body and helps to maintain optimum health. If done regularly, massage helps to regulate body functions physically, mentally, and spiritually. Listed below are few of the effects that massage has on the human body. Massage

- soothes and enables the nerves and pulse to function properly
- increases circulation of the blood and lymph so that waste material such as perspiration, urine, and excreta are discarded properly
- strengthens the lungs, intestines and other vital organs for proper functioning
- improves skin
- regulates the digestive system
- aids body in using fat deposits
- cures diseases such as paralysis and polio
- strengthens muscles and blood vessels
- helps athletes, gymnasts, and soldiers
- benefits people who are unable to do exercise
- strengthens bones by improving body efficiency and circulation
- relieves some problems and ailments people encounter in old age
- alleviates adhesions
- reduces swelling and thickening of tissues
- facilitates the assimilation of nutrients in food

For the Masseur/Masseuse

What requirements or conditions are essential for a masseur or masseuse to function at an optimum level? Massage is not an act of mere rubbing, a movement which may be useful to the skin but is useless to the muscles or organs beneath the skin. Massage helps to reach out well beneath the skin and soothe the internal organs of the body. This produces a state of relaxation and well-being.

Disposition. The masseur/masseuse should be of a calm and peaceful disposition. The act of massaging is an act of giving and, therefore, calls for a selfless attitude. Any mental disturbance or emotional upset may get transmitted to the patient through the sense of touch, causing discomfort to the patient. Therefore it is extremely important for the masseur/masseuse to be completely detached from his personal life and concentrate on giving maximum benefit to the patient. The masseur's/masseuse's hands should be warm to the touch. It is essential that the masseur or masseuse be free of any kind of disease and maintain strict personal hygiene. Hands should be washed with soap before starting with each patient and it is advisable to take a bath between patients. A fresh gown should be used for every patient.

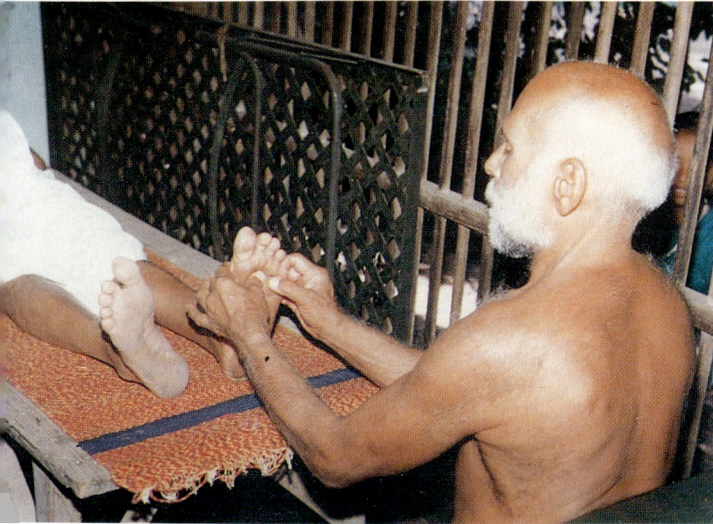

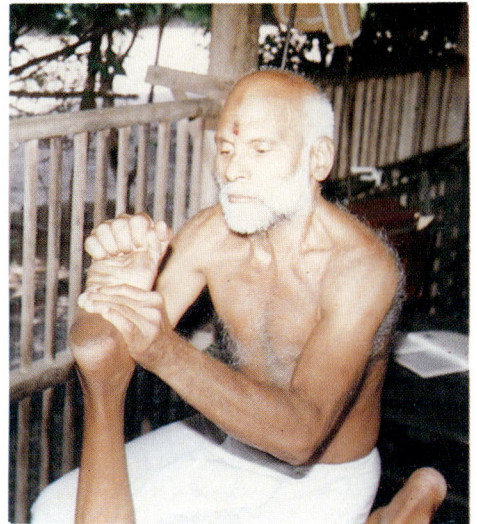

1. Sole (Feet) Massage 11. Foot Massage (Relaxation movement)

3. Foot Massage (Stretching)

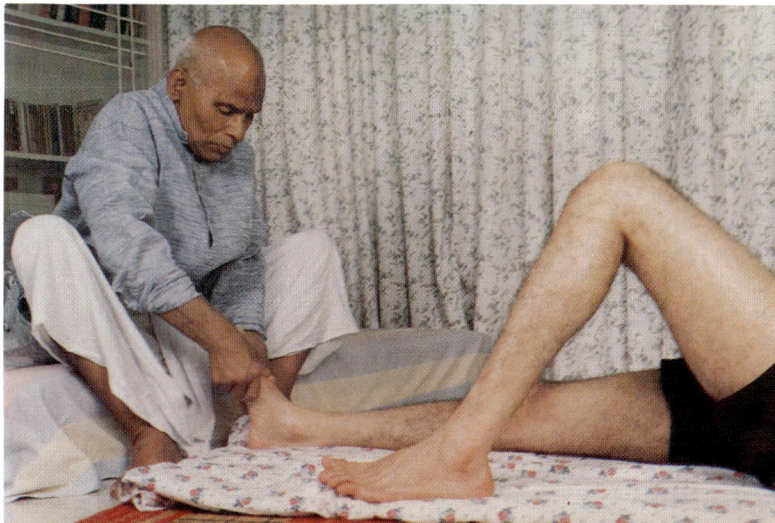

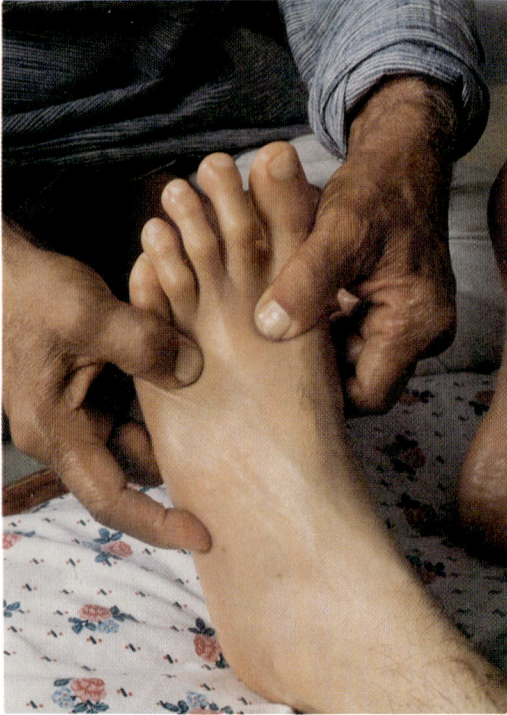

2.   Foot Massage (Pounding)

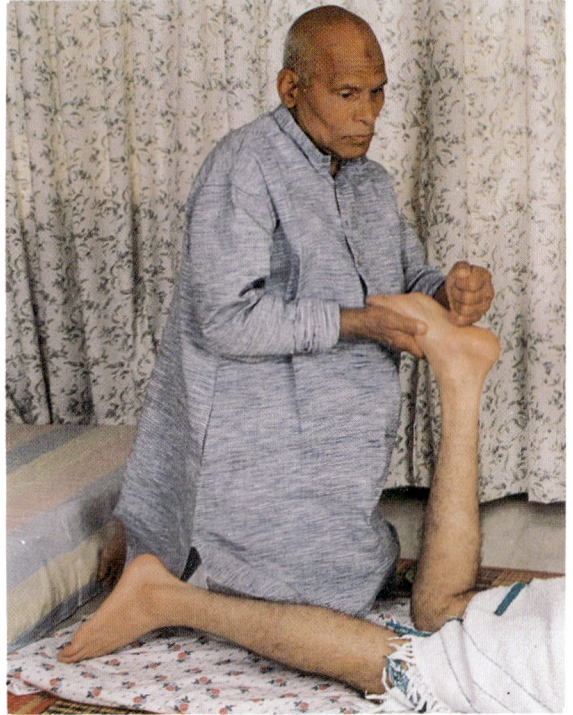

29.   Foot Massage (Beating)

5.   Knee Massage pressing the points

6.   Knee Massage for Arthritis

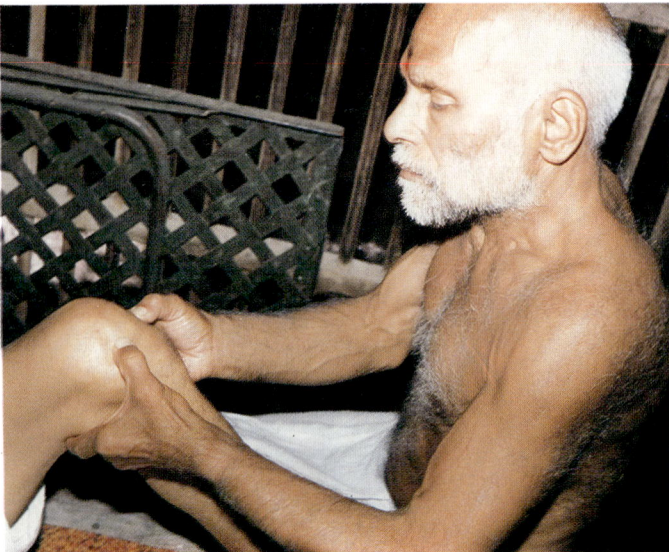

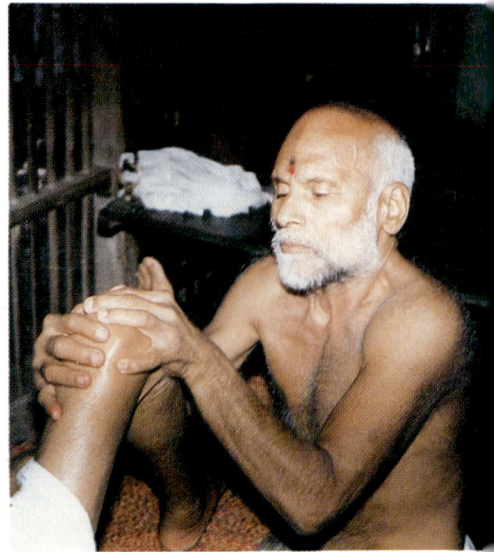

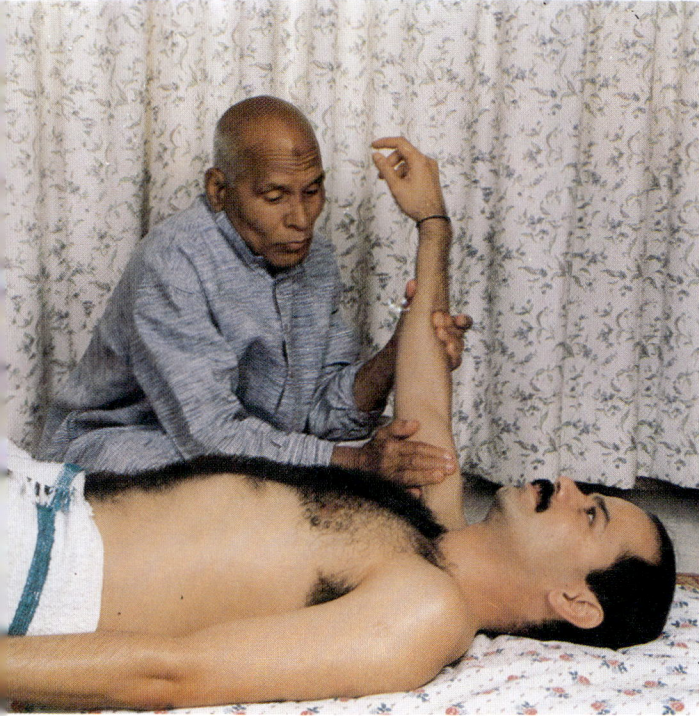

7. Arm Massage

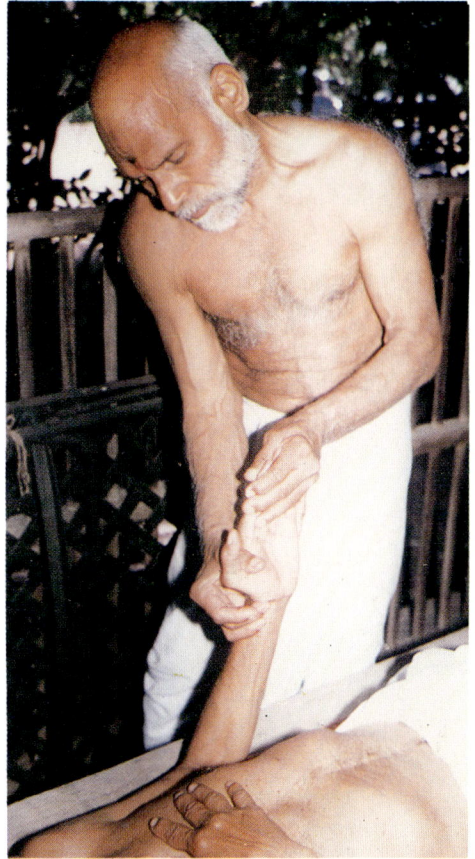

10. Palm Massage for removing tension

8. Palm Massage

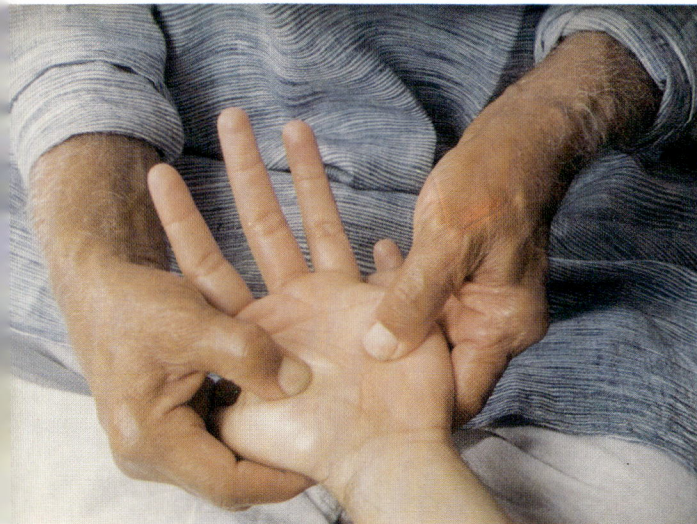

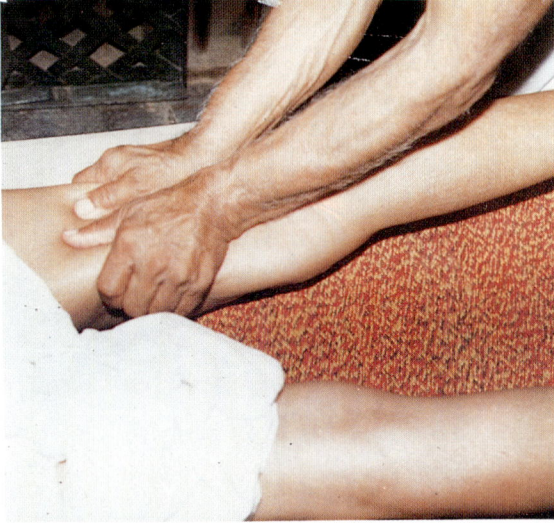

26. Upper Leg (Kneading) 27. Lower Leg (Kneading)

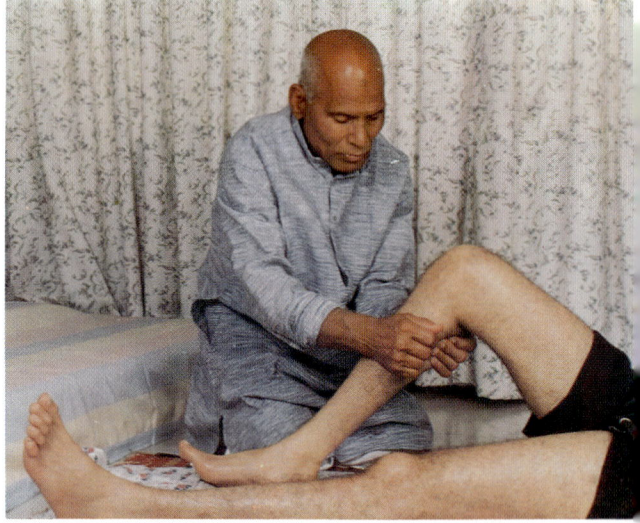

45. Massage during Pregnancy

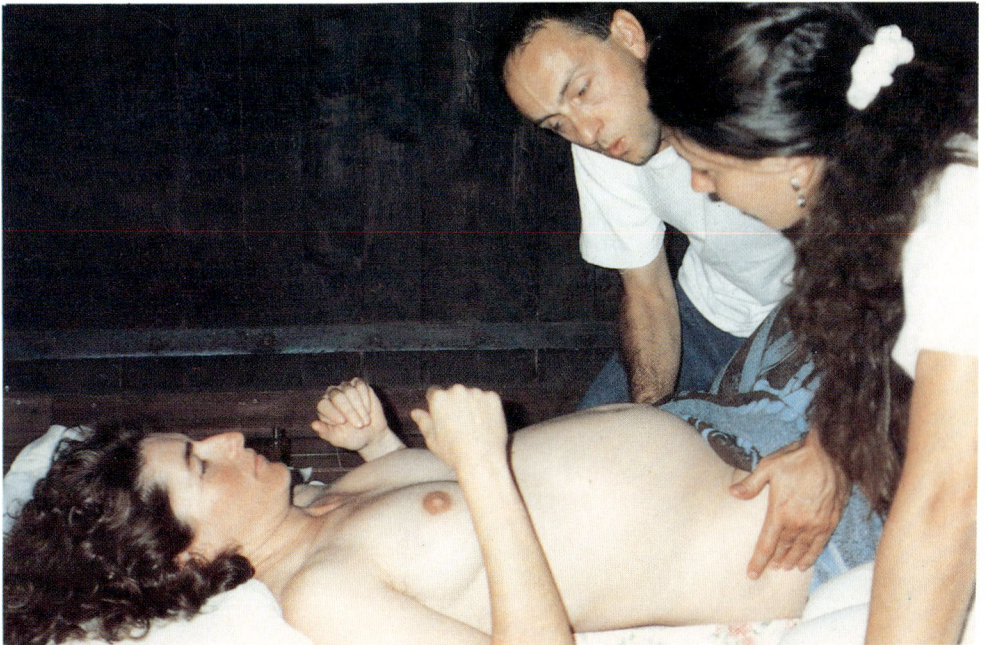

Setting. Select a comfortable place with enough light and ventilation. Depending on the season, the temperature of the room should be comfortable to the naked body. If possible, sunlight should seep into the room. Sometimes it is advisable for patients to sunbathe.

Massage Table. Because the massage table should support the whole body of the patient/client, it should have appropriate dimensions such as 7 feet by 2 feet or 6 feet by 2 feet. A thick sheet should be spread over it and should be changed for every patient.

Direction. Ask the patient to lie down on the massage table in a supine position. Massage of the head, neck and face is done in a sitting position. In cases of hot massage, rubbing causes friction and produces heat. Massage should start from the soles of the feet and move toward the heart. This enables the veins, which carry impure blood to the heart, to function better. In cases of cold massage, done with cold water or ice, the correct direction is from the head to the toes. Cold massage stimulates the arteries; in order to achieve appropriate stimulation, the temperature of the part being massaged should be lower than room temperature.

Duration. The duration of a massage will differ with the treatment. Generally a massage lasts for 30 to 45 minutes. In Ayurveda, the period for a general massage differs with the age of the patient. Newborn babies should be massaged for 15 minutes daily. Children up to the age of 4, 20 minutes. Youth and adults for 30 minutes, and old people for 40 minutes daily.

Process. The most suitable time for massage is early in the morning between 5 and 9 A.M. in the climate of India and evening between 4:30 and 6 P.M. For Westerners from 7:30 A.M. to 11:30 A.M. and 5 P.M. to 8 P.M. Apply oil before starting the squeezing technique. Massage all the areas of the body again with both hands. Use cross movements and squeeze all the muscles with bearable pressure. This helps to remove pain and tension from the extremities such as the toes and fingers. Squeeze the muscles until all the oil is absorbed by the skin. The joints of the fingers and toes should be rotated clockwise as well as anticlockwise to enhance the secretion of growth hormones. After squeezing, put a drop of oil on each nail so that the oil fills up the gap between the nail and the tissues around it. Oil massage yields maximum benefits if the patient is fasting. Massage the legs, arms, chest, abdomen, back, and hips, in that order.

Position and Pressure. Ask the patient to lie in a supine position for a body massage. Massage should be done slowly, but with sufficient pressure. Massage for a child should be done smoothly whereas for a gymnast, full pressure may be used. Apply pressure to the muscles while avoiding bones.

Medium. Normally oil is used for massage, but talcum powder is recommended for night-time massage.

Abdominal Massage. Massage of the abdomen should be done on an empty stomach. The patient's bladder should be empty before beginning the massage. Do not massage the abdomen unless the muscles are relaxed. Stop abdominal massage if the patient shows any signs of discomfort. Do not massage the abdomen for more than 5 minutes. In case the patient is suffering from heart disease or cerebral hemorrhage, do not massage the abdomen. Do not drag downwards on the navel. Do not massage anyone with intestinal ulcers.

For the Patient

The patient should be calm and relaxed. If the masseur/masseuse senses that the patient has any reservations or fears, he/she should help the patient to relax before starting the session. The massage session should start with breathing exercises, which should be repeated before abdominal massage. During winter, care should be taken to see that the patient does not get exposed to cold air. To aid this, the patient's body should be covered except for the portion that is being massaged. After a massage, bathing in cold water is beneficial. But if the patient is used to bathing in warm water, he/she may do so but after the warm bath, rub a cold wet towel over the body. After a bath the patient should be advised to lie down for about 10 minutes, covering the body. Once the massage is over, the patient should lie in *shavasana,* the corpse posture. The patient can concentrate on the eyebrow center, gradually moving the concentration to each part of the body, thus enabling the patient to relax completely.

For Women

During pregnancy or the menstrual cycle, massage the whole body except for the abdomen. While massaging the breasts, the sides should be massaged slowly and gently. After delivery, if the thighs, waist and abdomen are massaged well, the woman will more quickly regain her stamina, vigor and energy.

For Children

Ghee (butter made from cow's milk) massage is advised for children. Children should be massaged early in the morning. If possible, let the child remain in the tender sun rays for about 10 minutes. When a mother massages her baby, the communication through touch transmits a lot of love and affection. In case of any physical ailment, call an expert masseur/masseuse. After massage, use *petrissage* by grasping the muscles between the forefinger and the thumb and lifting them from the bone. Exercise all joints after massage.

Make ghee at home by boiling milk on a slow fire. After the milk comes to a boil, let it cool to room temperature. Add a little curd or yogurt to it. The curd (or yogurt) helps to ferment or curdle the milk. This curdled milk should then be churned until the butter and the butter milk separate easily. Heat the butter, which contains a small quantity of water, enough to melt it and bring to a boil. After the water evaporates the ghee emanates a sweet aroma, indicating that it is ready. See section on oils, pastes and essences for more information on ghee.

FOOT MASSAGE

Hold the foot, let it relax, then gently rub. Hold the side other than the one being rubbed.

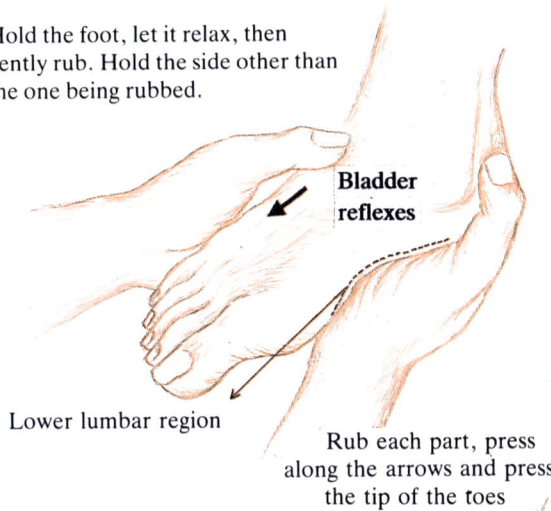

Bladder reflexes

Lower lumbar region

Rub each part, press along the arrows and press the tip of the toes

Fig. 9

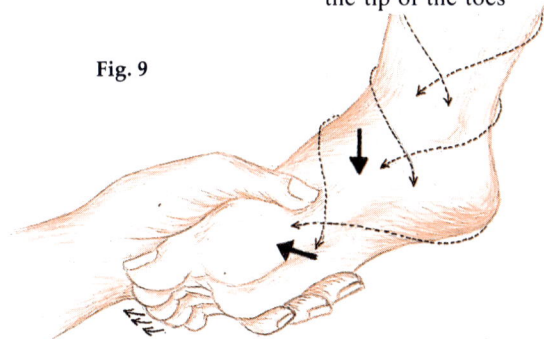

Massage with both hands at the end and squeeze the front part and take out every thin through toes

Guidelines

What general guidelines are helpful to a person who would like to practice massage? In order to energize the hands, the masseur/masseuse should relax them by shaking them gently, moving the wrists and palms in a circular manner or by mudras. Gradually increase the speed and move the hands faster until you feel a tingling sensation in the fingers. At this stage, the finger tips are charged with fresh energy.

In *Yoga Shastra* techniques certain postures and gestures are called *mudras*. They are forms of expression which help in communicating an idea. In the art of dance, the dancer uses different expressions like anger, joy, hatred, sadness, and astonishment. These are called Mukha Mudra, meaning expressions of the face. Hands and fingers are also used for gesticulating and communicating without talking. These are called Hasta Mudra, meaning expressions of the hands.

Feet. Ask the patient to lie on his/her back. Start with the feet. Shake and give vibrations to one of the feet. Using both hands, tap, and knead to shake the muscles of the feet on both sides of the muscles. Begin from the soles of the feet. Apply oil to the foot and sole and rub well. Press/pump all pressure points of the sole including the toes. Massage the right foot in a clockwise circular movement and the left foot in an anticlockwise direction. It is believed that diseases do not come near the person who massages his or her feet every night before going to bed.

Place the heel of the patient on the masseur's/masseuse's hand and hold the ankle joint with the thumb and other fingers (Figure 9). Press the tips of the toes (Photo 1). The reflexive points of the bladder and hip may be massaged well. The sole of the foot is very important because it is related with internal organs of the body (Photo 29). For reflexology or acupressure points please refer to Acupressure and Reflexology in Appendix A. Spiritual energy massage also has connection with some of those points. Put some oil on the nails and massage. Use pulling, pressing, and rubbing on the toes (Photo 2). The masseur/masseuse can then squeeze (Photo 11) the whole foot with both hands. Lastly, twist and pull each toe (Photo 3).

Lower Leg. When massaging the lower leg, have the patient keep his/her knee raised and bent, knead the muscles of the calves using oil and rubbing well. Place your thumbs on the lower part of the knee cap with the other fingers on the higher side of the knee cap (Photo 27). Press your fingers tightly near the tendons making circular movements with the thumbs. Rub the knee faster (Photo 6) and massage the lower leg so that the muscles of the calves loosen up completely. Give pressure to the points shown in Figure 10. Massage and rub both sides of the area of the ankle joint just above the heel.

Upper Leg and Knee. Tapping and kneading may be rendered to the upper

LOWER LEG MASSAGE

Fig. 10

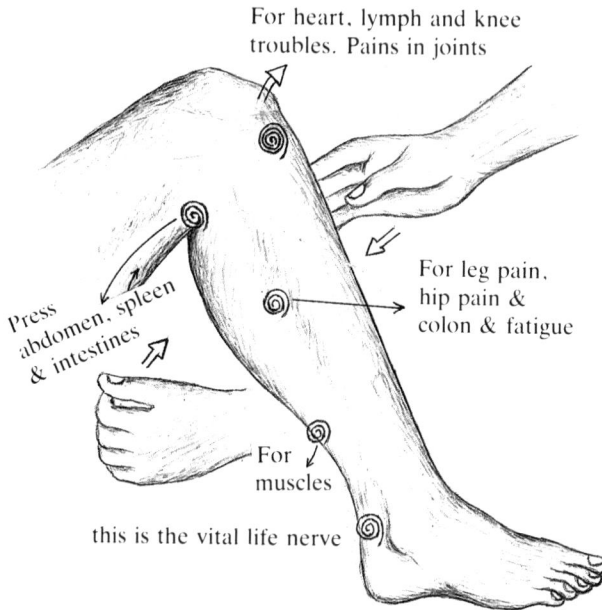

For heart, lymph and knee troubles. Pains in joints

For leg pain, hip pain & colon & fatigue

Press abdomen, spleen & intestines

For muscles

this is the vital life nerve

leg. Apply oil and rub the entire upper leg well. Massage the front of the thigh first. Remove muscular tension, which is the strongest in this area. Then massage the back of the thigh to stimulate the lymph nodes. Massage and stimulate the hollow portion of the knee (Photo 26). Figure 11 shows upper leg massage movements.

Ask the patient/client to stretch his/her leg. Shake the whole leg once again, causing vibration with your fingers. Finish the leg massage with a gentle touch. Repeat the same procedure for the other leg.

Knees. Pressing on the two hollow places (Photo 5) on the knee is for heart lymph and knee troubles. It also reduces the pain in front. Pressing on the back of the knee (2 points) is for abdomen, spleen and intestines. Rotating clockwise on the upper calf, outer side is for leg pain, colon and also for fatigue. Clockwise rotating on the lower calf outside is for muscles. Clockwise rotating on the ankles is to activise the vital life nerve.

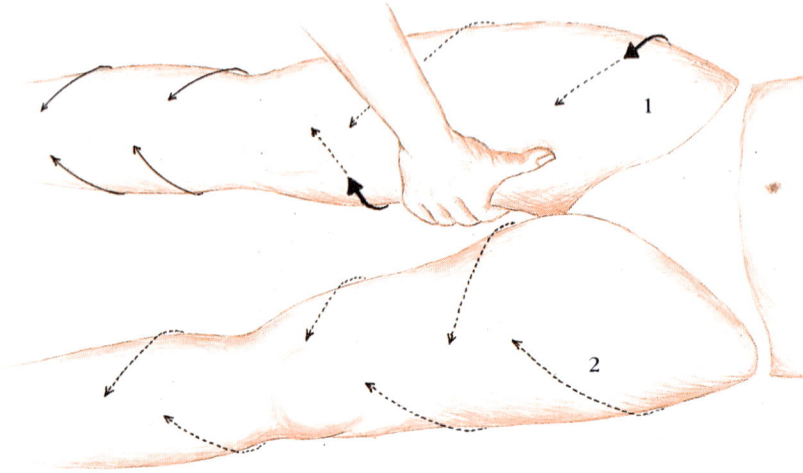

Fig. 11

UPPER LEG MASSAGE

1. Inguinal lymph nodes whose massage keeps colon in right
   shape and energizes the pelvic and hypogastric plexus.

2. Gentle rubbing excites sexual feelings. Hard pressing helps
   waist region and adductor and magnus. Helps circulation.
   Cures numbness. Increases sensitivity.

Arms. Shake the whole arm first and apply oil to the entire length, including
the palm and fingers. Looking at Figure 13 and Photo 7 will be helpful. Rub the
whole arm with pressure. With a circular movement, excite the lymph nodes in the
upper arm. Knead and press the muscles of the upper arm. Wringing can also be
rendered. Apply oil in the armpit, press the center of the armpit until you feel
pulsation.

Stimulate the lymph nodes in the hollow of the elbow from both sides with
your fingers. Do this on the side of the bone as well as in the hollow of the joint. Block
the lower arm with the thumb in the hollow of the elbow with your fingers on the
bone. With sufficient pressure, bring the thumb down the length of the lower arm.
Massage the whole arm again (Figure 12). Massage the palm and press the inside of
the palm (Photo 8). Massage the nails with oil along with the fingers. Pull each finger
and shake the whole hand (Photo 10). Repeat the same procedure for the other arm.

Pressing (pumping) on the index and the middle fingers together helps to
gain one-pointedness. Locking the index and the thumb tips together helps to cure
nervousness.

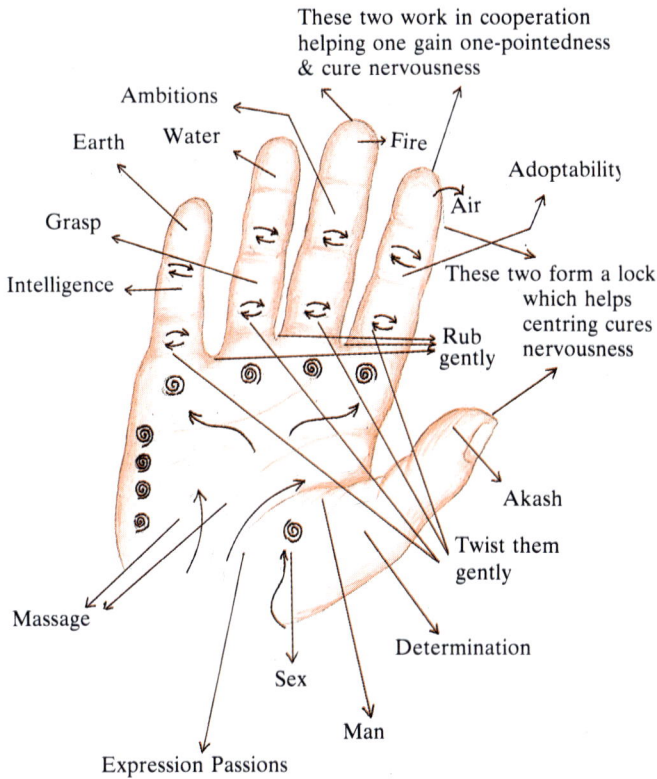

These two work in cooperation helping one gain one-pointedness & cure nervousness

Ambitions

Earth   Water

Fire

Adoptability

Air

Grasp

These two form a lock which helps centring cures nervousness

Intelligence

Rub gently

Akash

Twist them gently

Massage

Determination

Sex

Man

Expression Passions

Fig. 12

PALM MASSAGE

Abdomen. The navel is a very important part of the body because 72,000 nerve centers converge there. The fetus in a mother's womb is connected by these nerve endings. All vital fluids flow from the mother to the child through this channel. Before starting abdominal massage, place the middle finger in the hollow depth of the navel to check the pulsation of the patient/client. If you do not feel pulsation, the patient may have a stomach ailment. Pour a little oil in the navel. This area has many lymph nodes. A clockwise circular movement starting at the navel can help to regulate the circulation of digestive fluids. Apply oil to the entire abdomen and massage it from right to left exerting some pressure. Press on both sides at the point where the rib cage ends as shown in Photos 45A, 45. On the right is the liver and on the left the stomach. If the patient/client has any pain on either of these sides, massage gently, or stop depending on what feedback you are getting from the

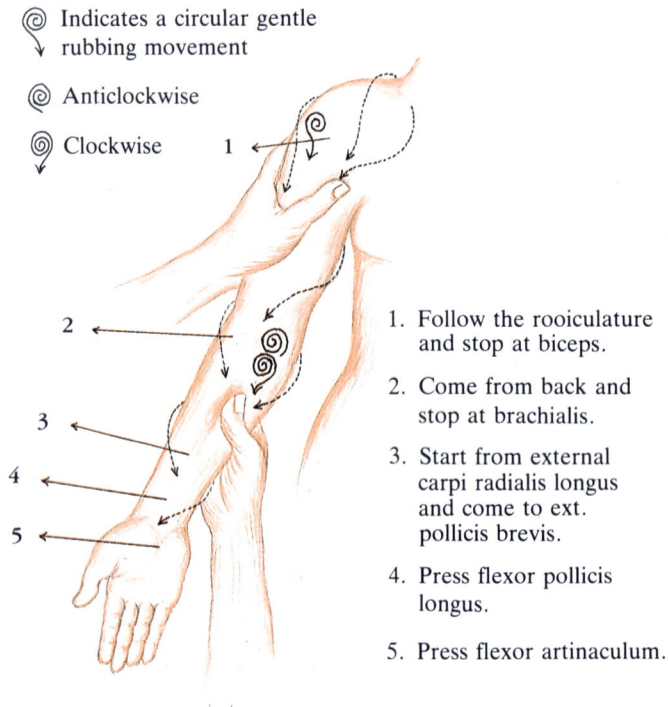

@ Indicates a circular gentle
↓ rubbing movement

@ Anticlockwise

@ Clockwise

1. Follow the rooiculature and stop at biceps.

2. Come from back and stop at brachialis.

3. Start from external carpi radialis longus and come to ext. pollicis brevis.

4. Press flexor pollicis longus.

5. Press flexor artinaculum.

ARM MASSAGE   Fig. 13

patient/client. Otherwise, give circular massage around the navel starting with small circles. End the massage gently after rendering vibrations with the fingers.

In the case of pregnant ladies abdomen massage should be done very gently by the masseuse or her husband. It helps normal deliyery.

Chest. Spread oil evenly on the entire area of the chest. Figure 15 shows the motions for front body massage. Massage the rib cage and the top of the chest with circular movements. When massaging the breasts begin with big circular movements and gradually make smaller circles near the nipples. This gives a proper shape to the breasts. With both men and women pull the nipples gently yet tightly; this will energize all the capillaries of the blood vascular system and increase the circulation of lymphatic system. A network of lymph modes is found in this area. Finish the chest massage with a gentle touch.

Waist. Ask the patient to lie on his left side with his left leg straight and the

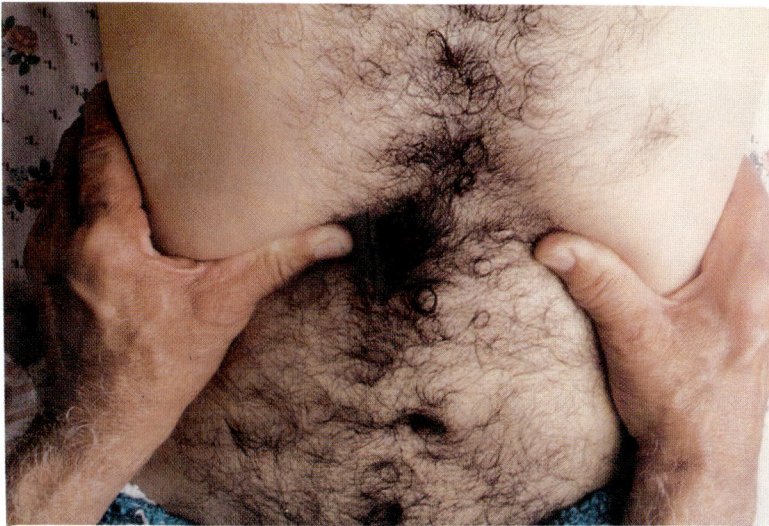

45a. Abdomen rib cage Massage

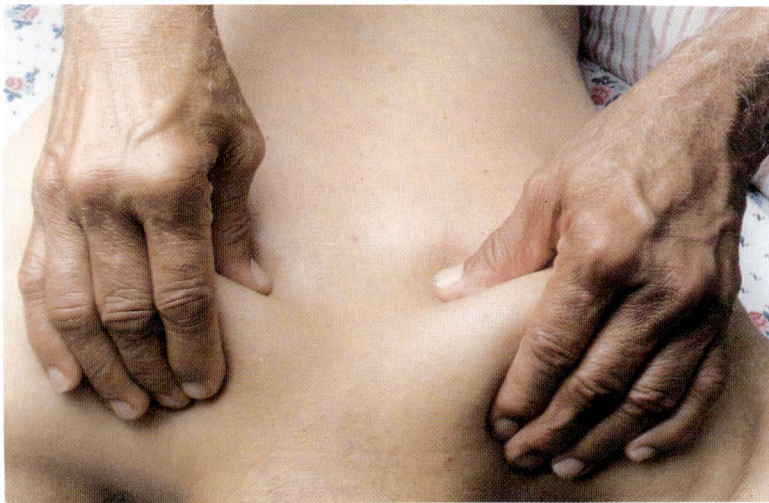

37.   Back Massage (Rolling)

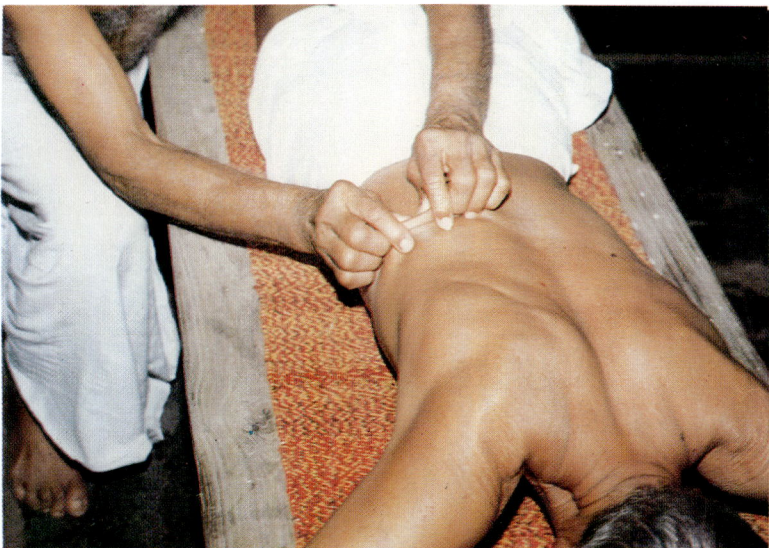

30.   Beating for Back Massage

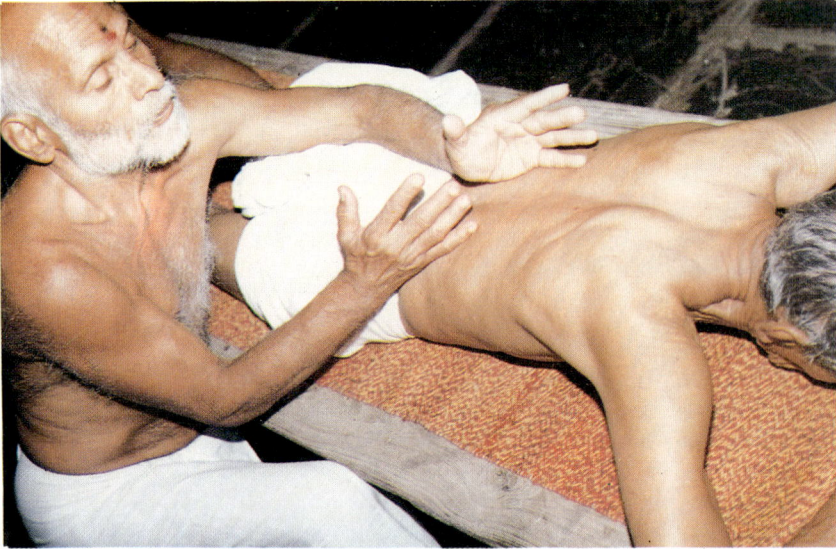
36.   Back Massage (Hacking)

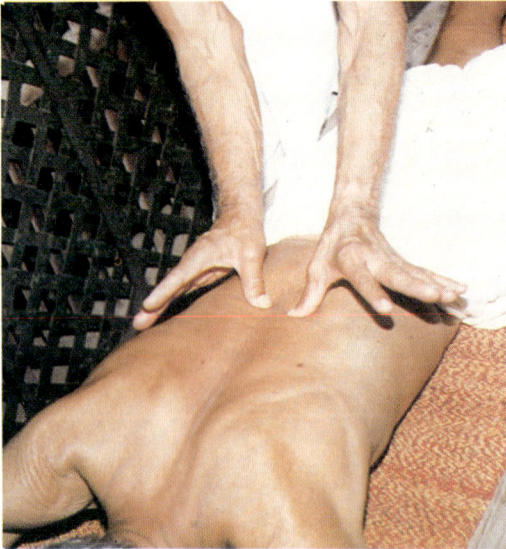
35.   Back Massage both sides of the spine

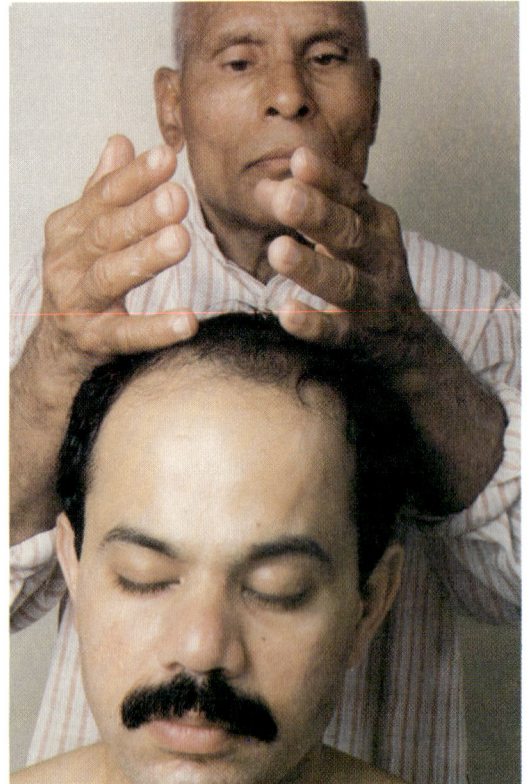
9.   Head Massage

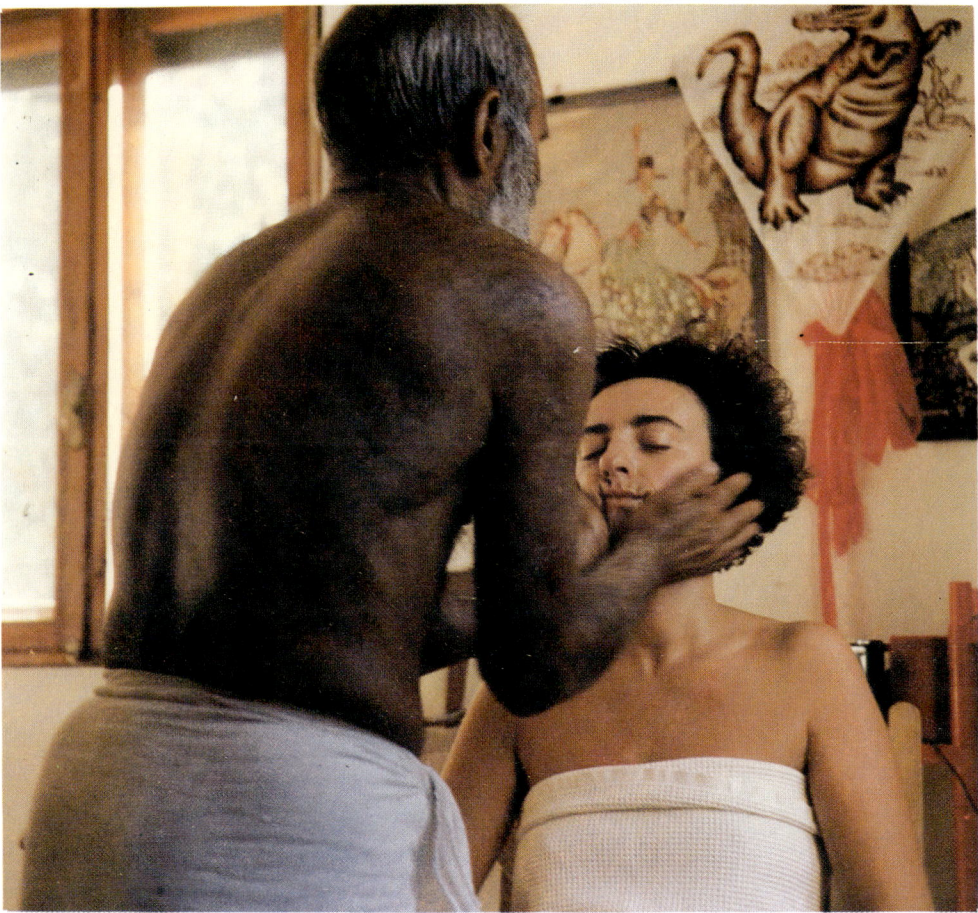
12.   Massaging Cheeks (Front)

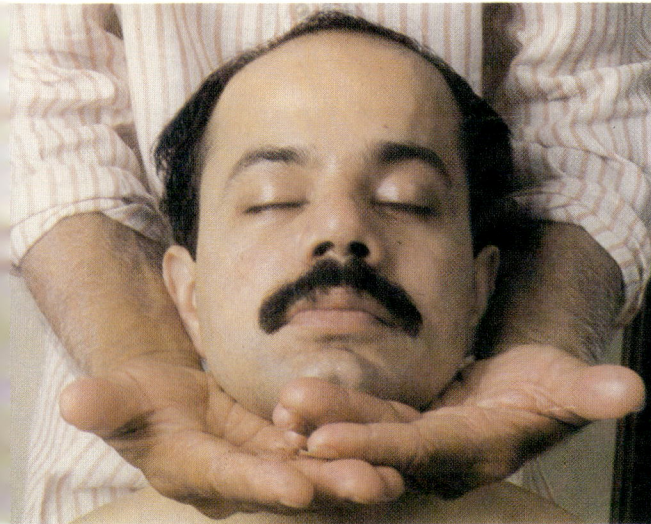
14.   Massaging the Jaw

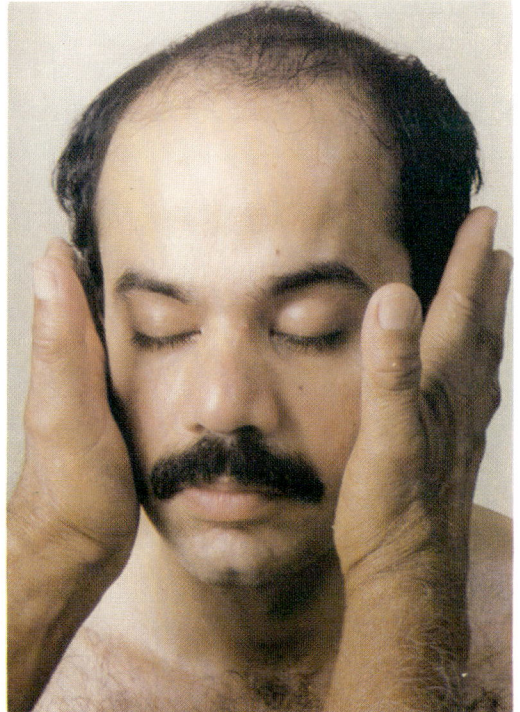
13.   Massaging the Cheeks

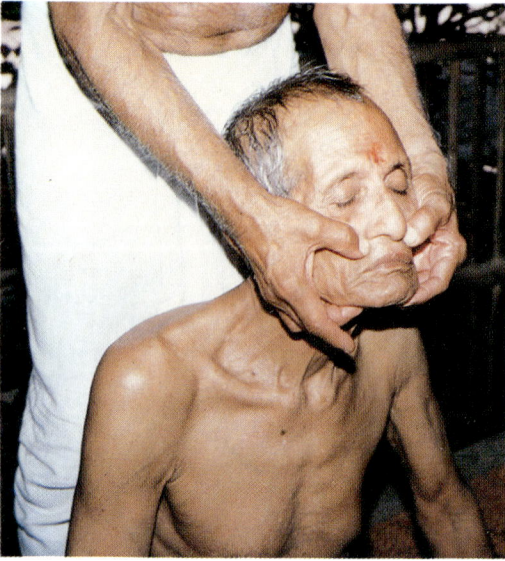

15.   Face Massage points below the cheek
       bones

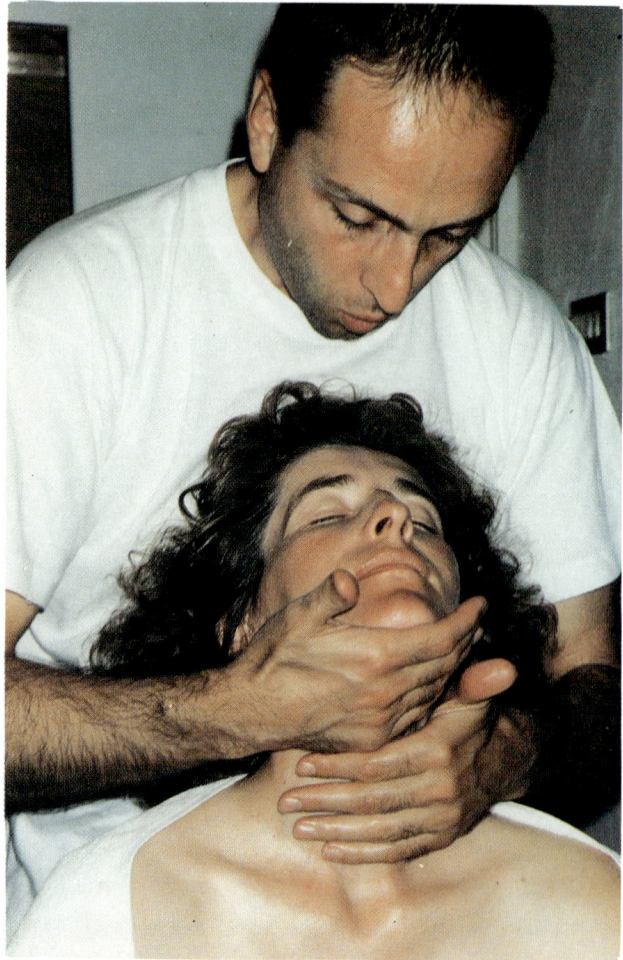

17.   Neck Massage

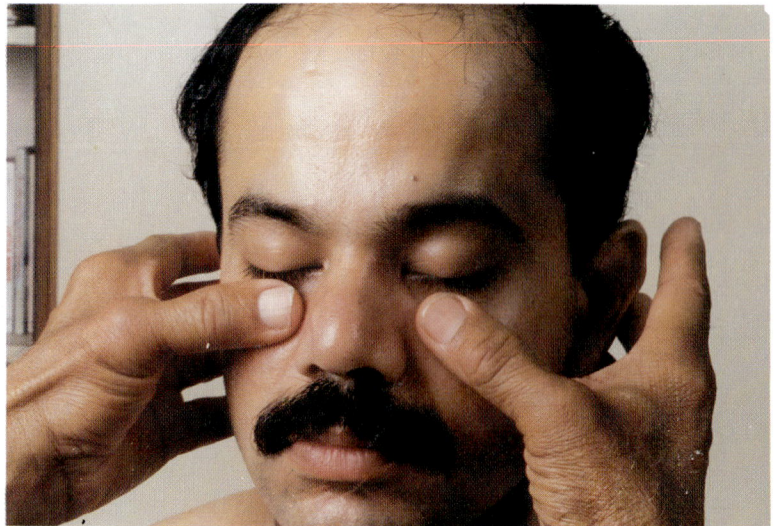

16.   Massaging the Eyes

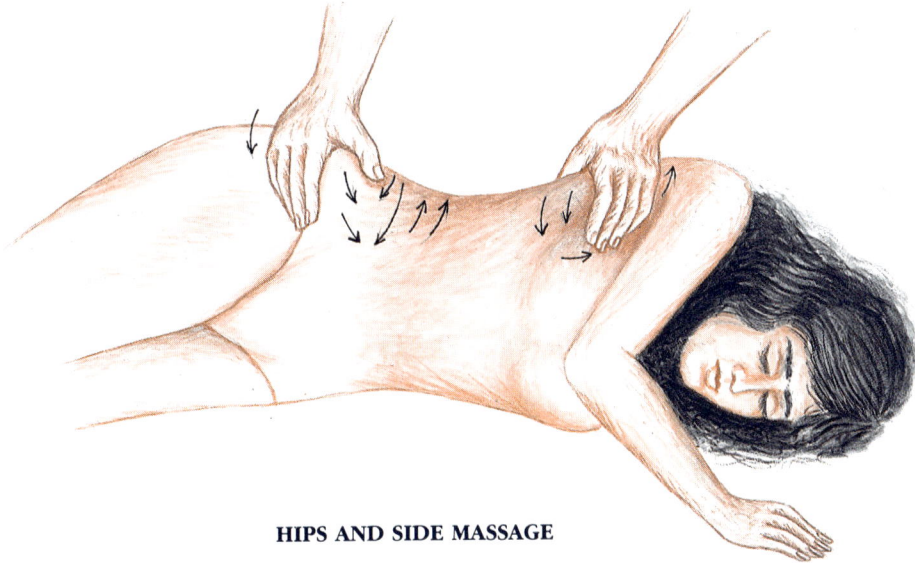

HIPS AND SIDE MASSAGE

Fig. 14

This massage helps stomach, intestine, waist region, pelvic plexus,
hypogastric plexus, colon, liver, spleen, and all tensions.
It is very relaxing and energizing.

right leg slightly bent as shown in Figure 14. While sitting behind the patient,
massage the waist, lumbar region, and the ribs on the side. Then move your hands
simultaneously. Move one hand in a clockwise direction and the other in an
anticlockwise direction as illustrated in the figure. Repeat the procedure on the
other side also. This massage helps the waist to become more flexible.

Back. Have the patient/client lie down on his/her stomach for back massage.
According to Kundalini Shastra in yoga, human beings have seven *chakras* along the
spine which are centers of consciousness. Details of these chakras may be found in
the section on chakras. In order to manipulate these centers, the masseur should
locate these areas and points along the vertebral column. Put oil in these areas and
massage them with your thumbs using circular movements (Photo 35). Placing the
thumbs at the base of the spine, move the hands upward while making semicircular
movements on the whole back and on both sides of the spine. While doing this keep
both the thumbs on either side of the vertebral column as shown in Figures 16 &
17. Tapping and kneading are appropriate. Apply bearable pressure while rubbing.
The recipient may keep his arms under his forehead during this back massage. Oil
the spine and massage it from the base to the top (Photo 30). Lift the skin on the
back with the thumb and forefinger (Photo 37). If the skin does not get lifted

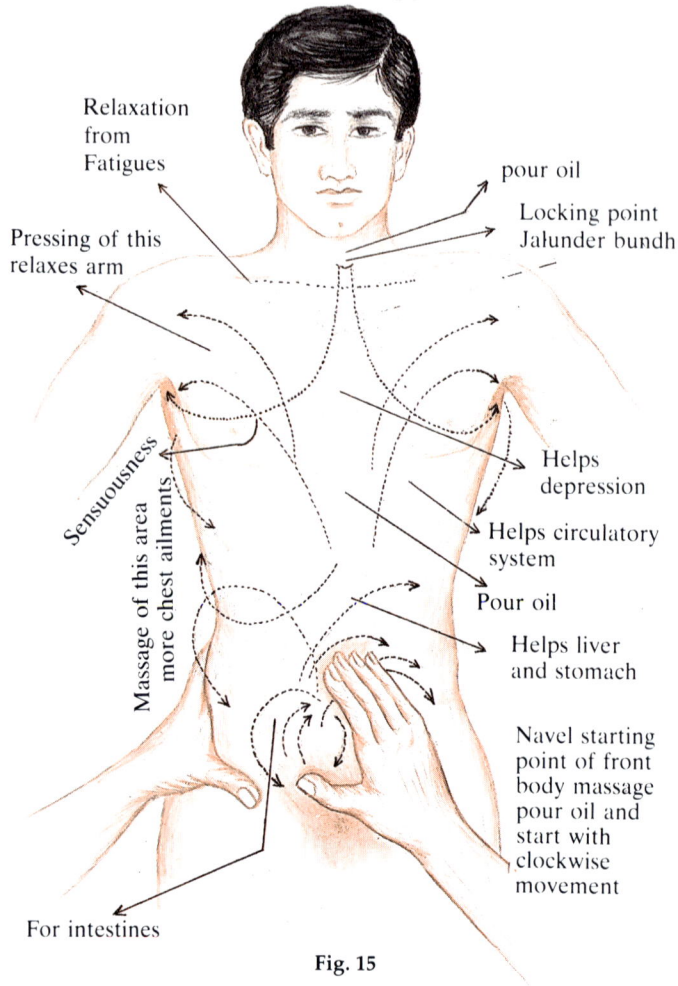

Relaxation
from
Fatigues

pour oil

Locking point
Jalunder bundh

Pressing of this
relaxes arm

Sensuousness

Massage of this area
more chest ailments

Helps
depression

Helps circulatory
system

Pour oil

Helps liver
and stomach

Navel starting
point of front
body massage
pour oil and
start with
clockwise
movement

For intestines

Fig. 15

FRONT BODY MASSAGE

properly, a corresponding internal organ may not be functioning properly. To
rectify this problem give more vibration and stroking (Photo 36) to the entire area
of the back. And with a gentle touch finish the massage of the back.

Head, Neck, and Face. The human body has ten gates, namely, the anus,
genitals, the mouth, two nostrils, two eyes, two ears, and the brahma randhra
(situated at the top of the cranium). The brahma randhra is on the head at the width
of eight fingers from the middle of the eyebrows. The brahma randhra provides

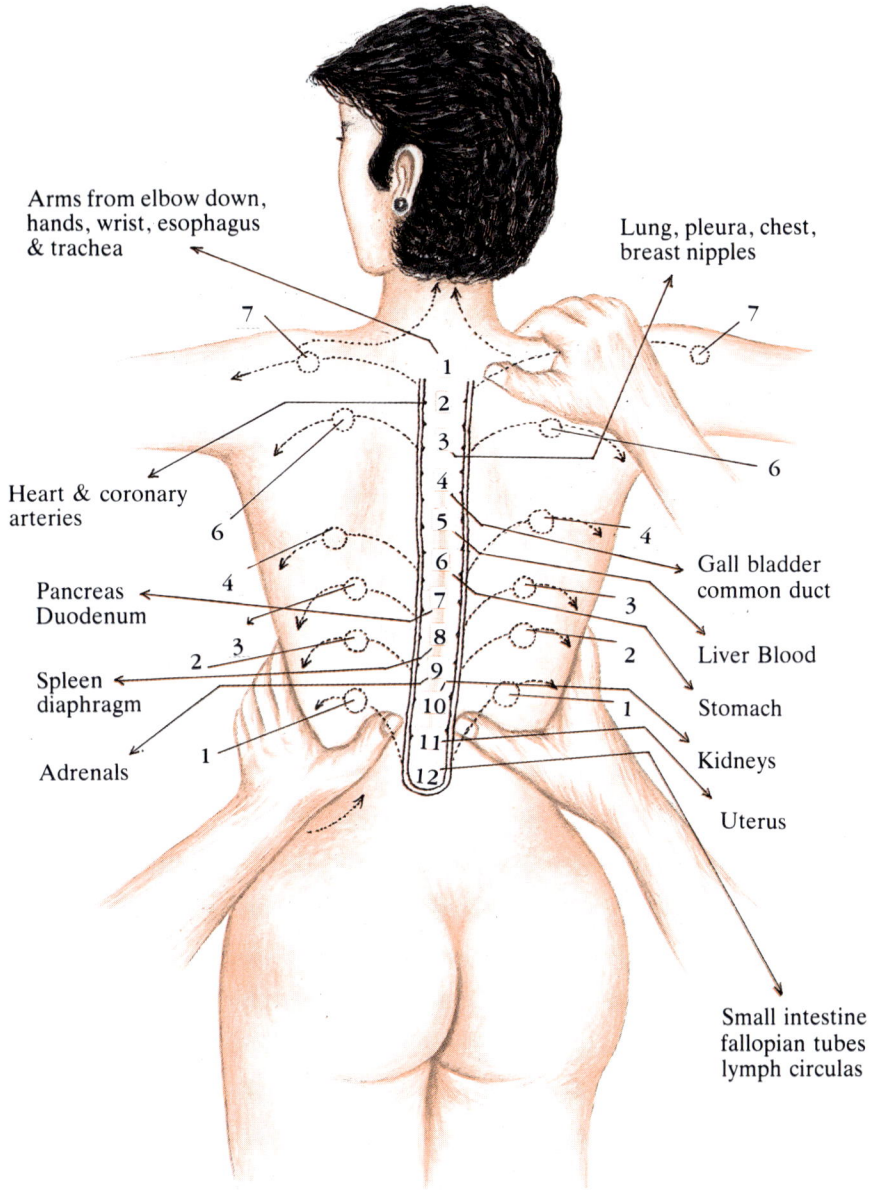

Arms from elbow down,
hands, wrist, esophagus
& trachea

Lung, pleura, chest,
breast nipples

7

7

1

2

3

4

5

6

Heart & coronary
arteries

6

Gall bladder
common duct

4

4

Pancreas
Duodenum

7

3

Liver Blood

8

2

3

9

2

Spleen
diaphragm

10

1

Stomach

1

11

Kidneys

Adrenals

12

Uterus

Small intestine
fallopian tubes
lymph circulas

UPPER BACK MASSAGE

Fig. 16

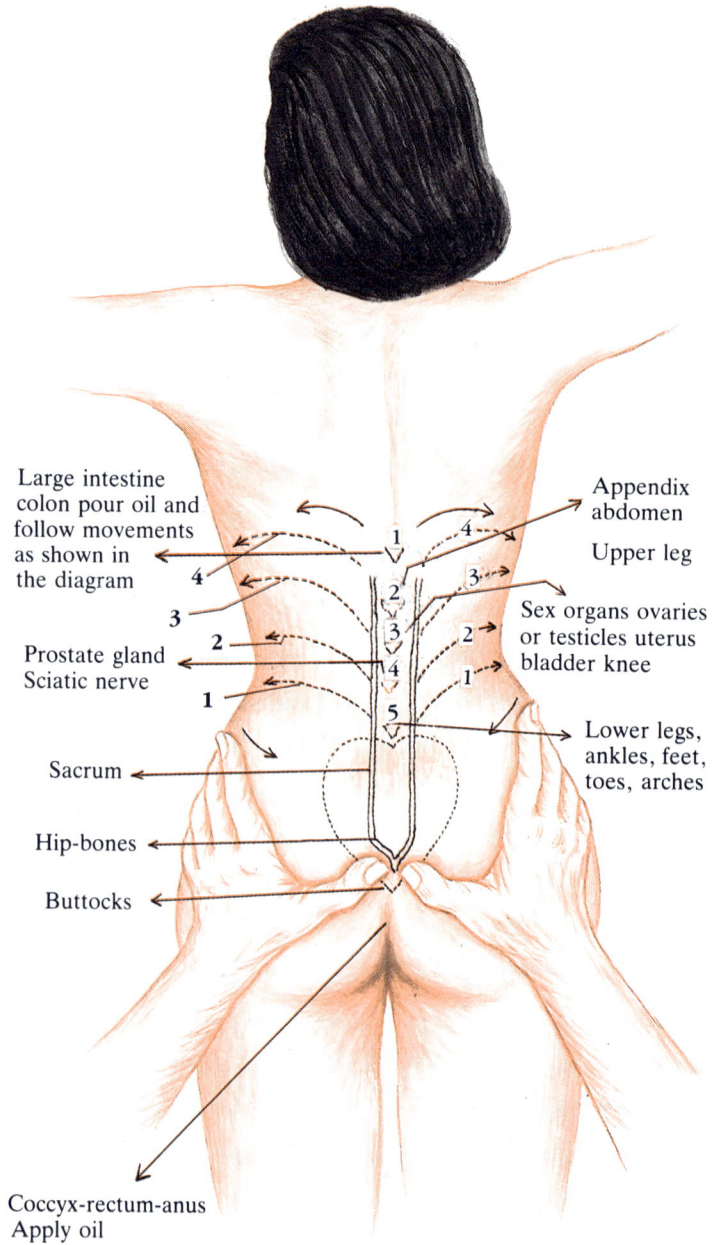

Large intestine
colon pour oil and
follow movements
as shown in
the diagram

Appendix
abdomen

Upper leg

Prostate gland
Sciatic nerve

Sex organs ovaries
or testicles uterus
bladder knee

Sacrum

Lower legs,
ankles, feet,
toes, arches

Hip-bones

Buttocks

Coccyx-rectum-anus
Apply oil

LOWER BACK MASSAGE

Fig. 17

1. Base of the spine – Seat of Muladhara
2. End of the hip bone – Seat of Swadhishthana
3. End of the rib cage – Seat of surya
4. End of the shoulder blades – Seat of Anahata
5. End of collar bone – Seat of Vishudha

HEAD MASSAGE

Fig. 18

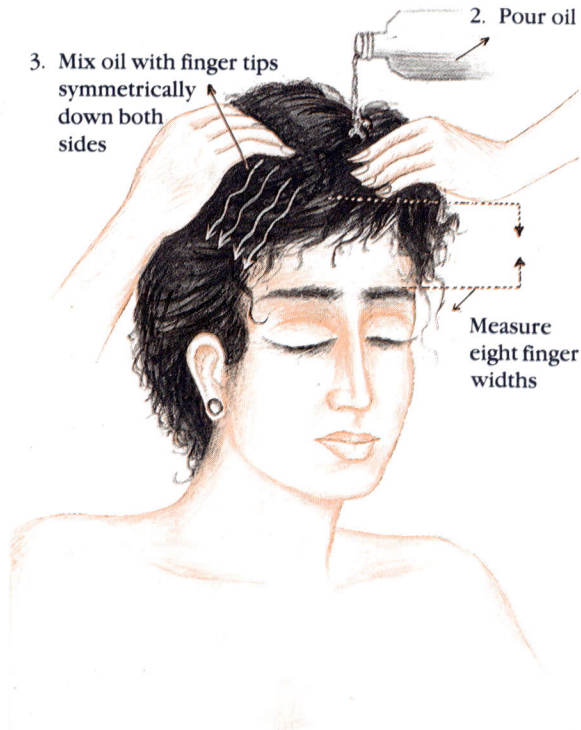

2. Pour oil

3. Mix oil with finger tips symmetrically down both sides

Measure eight finger widths

energy to the fetus. Eight gates out of the ten are above the neck, therefore the head is very important.

Do head and neck massage while the patient/client is in a sitting position as shown in Photo 12. Face massage may also be done with the patient lying down as in Photo 20. Start with the face by applying oil. Next massage the cheeks with both the hands using a circular movement. Massage the neck and the collar bone. Wringing (Photo 17) can be used on the neck. Massage the jaws (Photo 14), chin, lips and nose (Photos 15 & 18). Make circular movements with the thumb in the eyebrow area and around the eyes simultaneously. Apply pressure near the ears (Photo 19). Massage the forehead. Rub gently on the scalp and clap. Put a drop of oil into each ear and ask the receiver to move his lower jaw so that the drop of the oil may enter the ear. Dip the forefinger into the oil and apply inside each nostril.

HEAD MASSAGE

Fig. 19

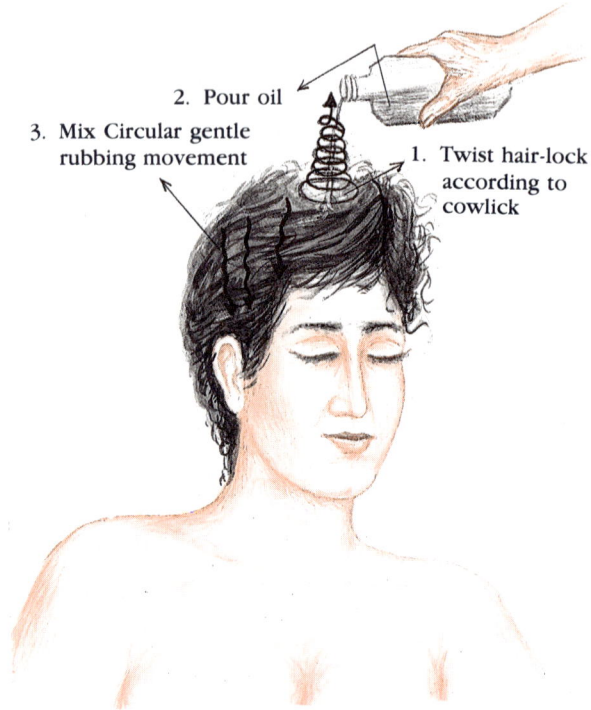

2. Pour oil

3. Mix Circular gentle
   rubbing movement

1. Twist hair-lock
   according to
   cowlick

If you have pure rose water, you may wish to put a drop in each eye. Photo 16 shows eye massage.

If nourishing oils are applied on the cranium at least for a period of nine months after the child is born, the child will receive more energy with which to think, learn and remember. That child is likely to have good eyesight for the rest of its life. Head massage during this period strengthens the nervous system. Oil applied to the head is absorbed into the roots of the hair which are connected by nerve fibers to the brain. Oil combined with massage strengthens and nourishes the hair and reduces dryness. Morning is a very good time for head massage. Applying sandalwood paste on the forehead is very good for the brain. It helps one to meditate and relax.

Massage of the eyebrows relaxes the whole body and is very therapeutic for the eyes and their nerves. Massage of the forehead improves sight and power of

HEAD MASSAGE

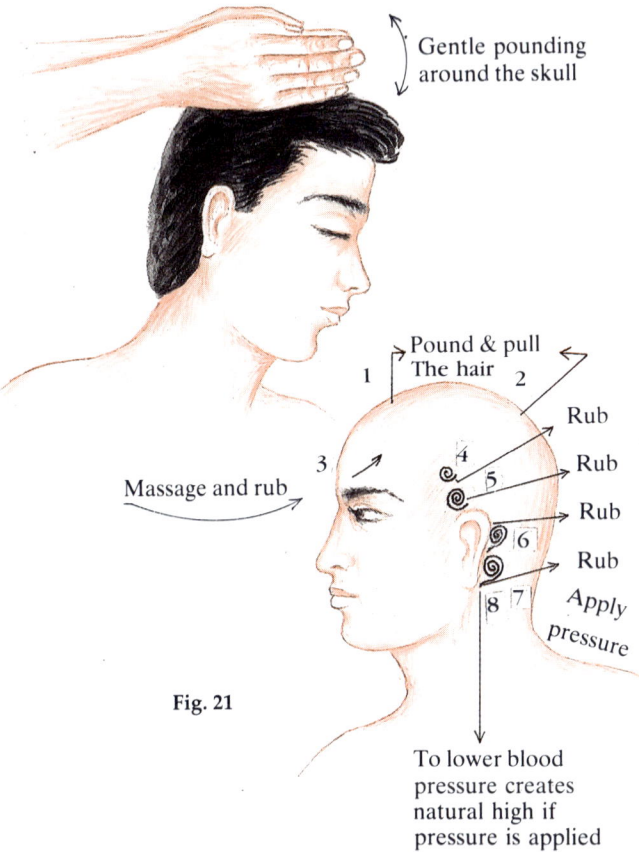

Gentle pounding around the skull

Pound & pull The hair

1

2

3 Massage and rub

Rub

Rub

Rub

Rub

Apply pressure

To lower blood pressure creates natural high if pressure is applied

Fig. 21

HEAD MASSAGE

Massage Following the Arrows

Fig. 20

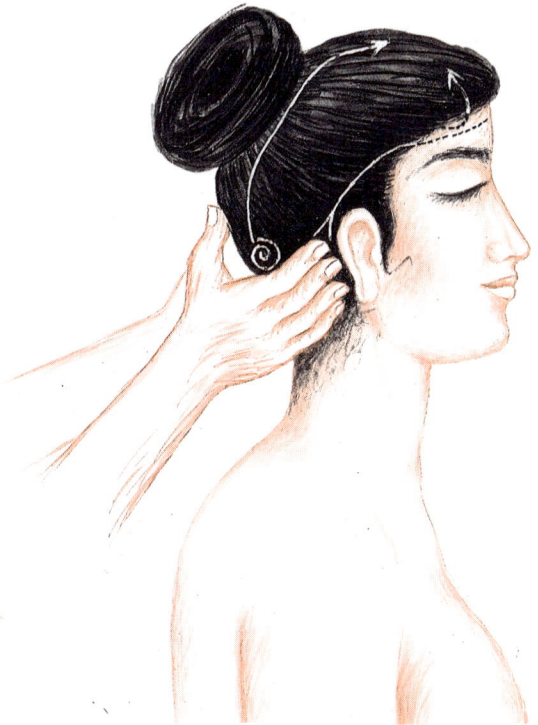

concentration. Head massage also increases the oxygen supply to the brain along with the circulation of the cerebrospinal fluid. It also increases the level of life energy. Scalp massage cures dryness, loss of hair, and premature baldness.

Three important points on the head are the brahma randhra, the crest area (the spot of the *shikha* or choti, which is the whorl at the top of the head) and the medulla oblongata (Figures 18-21) (the beginning of the brain stem or the place where the neck meets the skull). Pour oil on the three points, one after another. Spread the oil evenly and press the medulla oblongata; bring the fingers toward the forehead along the sides of the ears. Pound the head with both hands to energize the finer capillaries for circulation. Rub the three above-mentioned points. Press the skull (Photo 23) with both hands. Twist the hair on all the three points and pull gently. Give vibration with fingers of both hands (Photos 9 & 24) and finish the massage with a gentle touch. Photos 21 to 23 show a number of massage techniques for the head.

By massaging the brain stem the flow of cerebrospinal fluid increases. Twisting the whorl at the top of the head and the crest area and massaging those areas creates alertness and improves memory. Massaging the pineal gland area stimulates stomach and lower legs. Rubbing point 4 (in Figure 21) improves sight and helps lungs and heart functioning. Rubbing point 5 helps to balance the humor of wind in colon and intestines. Rubbing point 6 is good for brain and ears, and point 8 gives stability. Giving pressure on point 7 balances gas and nervous system.

COLD MASSAGE

Since cold massage stimulates the arteries, begin with the head and move downward to the soles of the feet. Do not, as a rule, expose the whole body of the patient/client except the particular area or limb that is being massaged. In some cases use ice or ice-cold water. You will need two towels, one for the cold water and the other for drying. Squeeze the water from the wet towel, fold it lengthwise and wind it around the right palm. Ask the patient to sit so that the masseur/masseuse can start massaging from the head and move down to the neck, face and shoulders. Immediately after the cold massage, rub the head with the dry towel. Now ask the patient to lie face down so that the back, including the buttocks, can be massaged. Rub the back with a dry towel after massaging. When the patient lies on his/her back, cold massage may be given to the chest, abdomen, hands, legs, and soles consecutively. Rub the areas with the dry towel after the massage.

After a cold massage, give a soft massage with warm hands or apply talcum powder. Employ gentle stroking, tapping, wringing, clapping, and very gentle friction. Because cold massage helps to dissolve body fat, it is advisable to give this treatment to overweight patients. This massage is also beneficial for those suffering from skin diseases. The patient/client should rest for 30 minutes after a cold massage. Be sure the patient/client is warm enough to be comfortable.

BEAUTY MASSAGE FOR WOMEN AND MEN

Massage adds a glaze to the skin and increases beauty. Regular massage of the face and body slows down the effects, thereby maximizing one's youth and energy. When problems, disease, and other factors destroy the natural rhythm of the body and when the body becomes dry, ugly, rough, heavy, thin, and so on, certain types of massage can create miracles. If old men and women undergo 40 days of massage every year, they will look younger than their age. If one follows the instructions regarding food, work, and sleep, during and after the prescribed 40 days, some signs of old age may be erased.

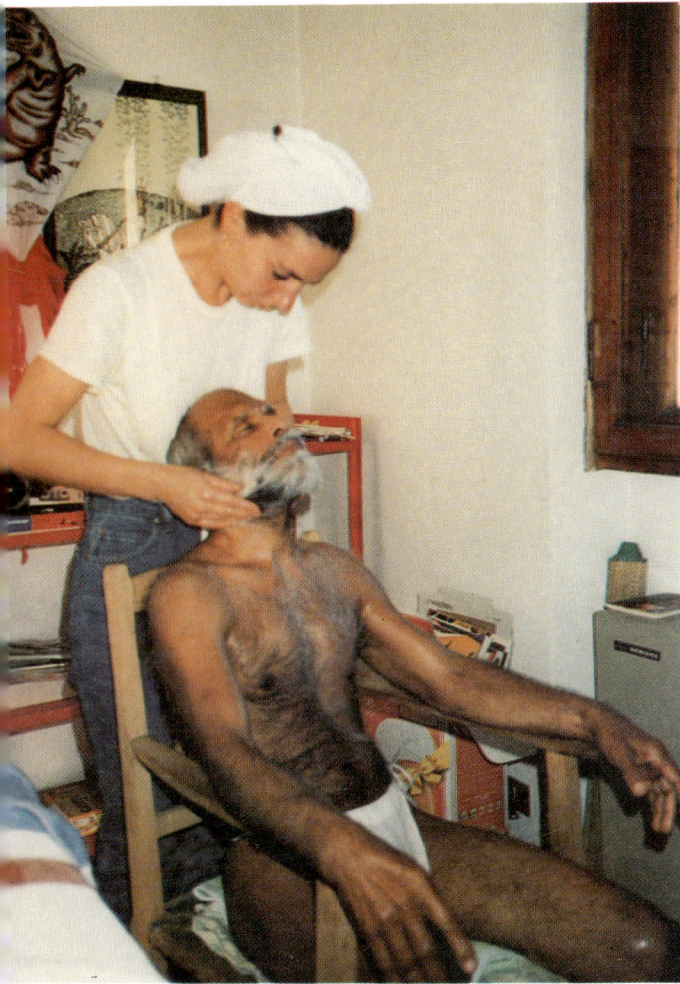

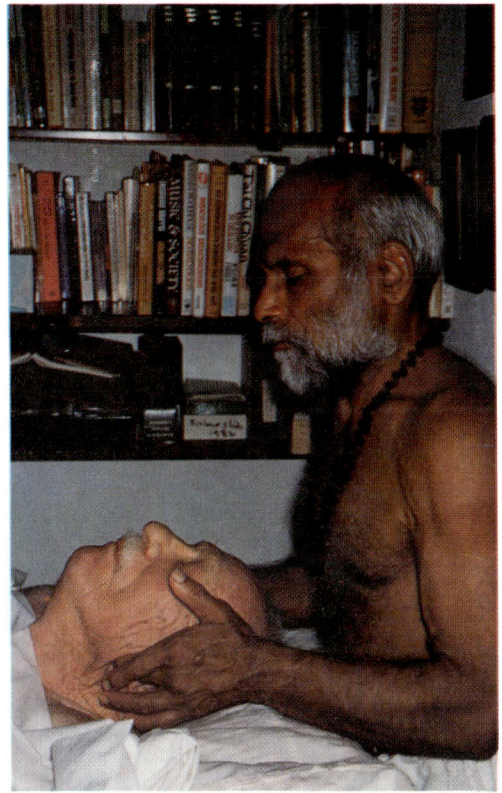

20. Face Massage

18. Face Massage

19. Ear Massage points below and behind the ears

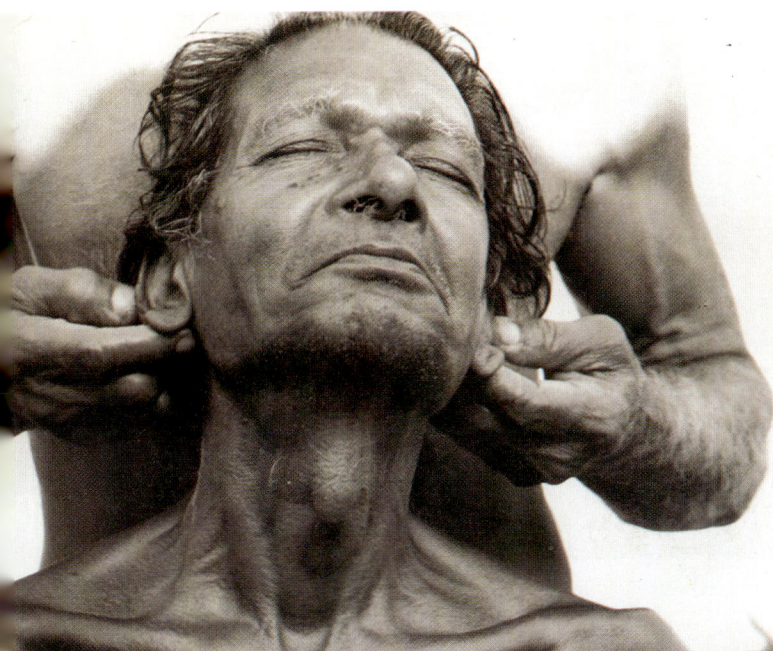

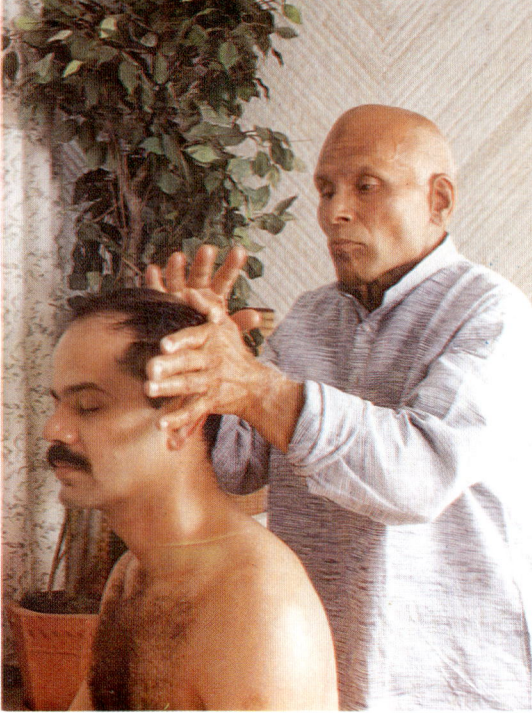

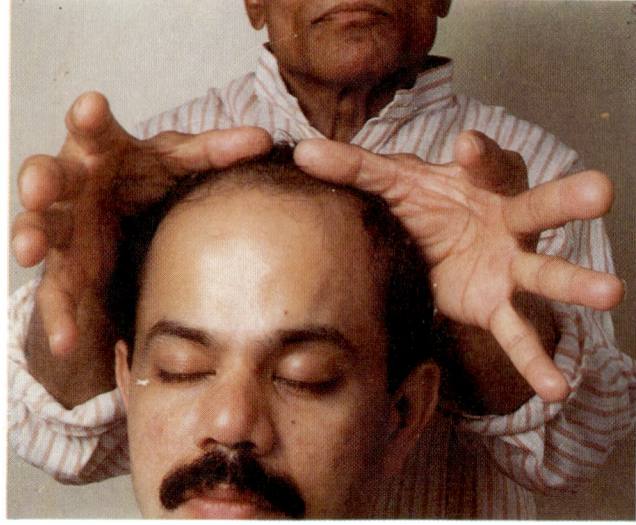

25. Head Massage from behind the ears to Brahma Randhra

22. Head Massage

24. Head Massage (Digital Vibrations)

23. Head Massage

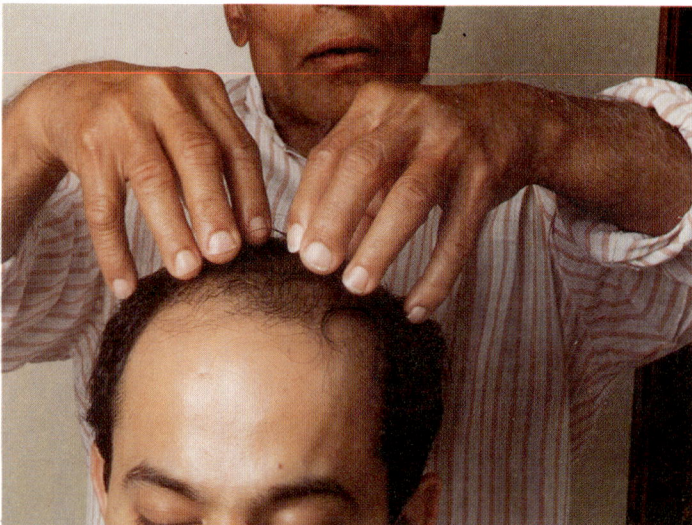

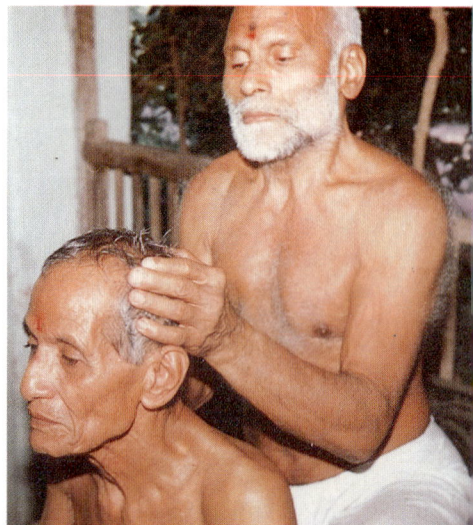

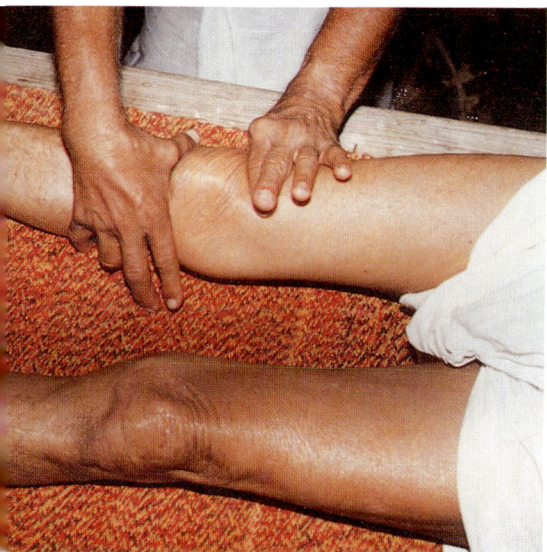

Knee Massage (Wringing)

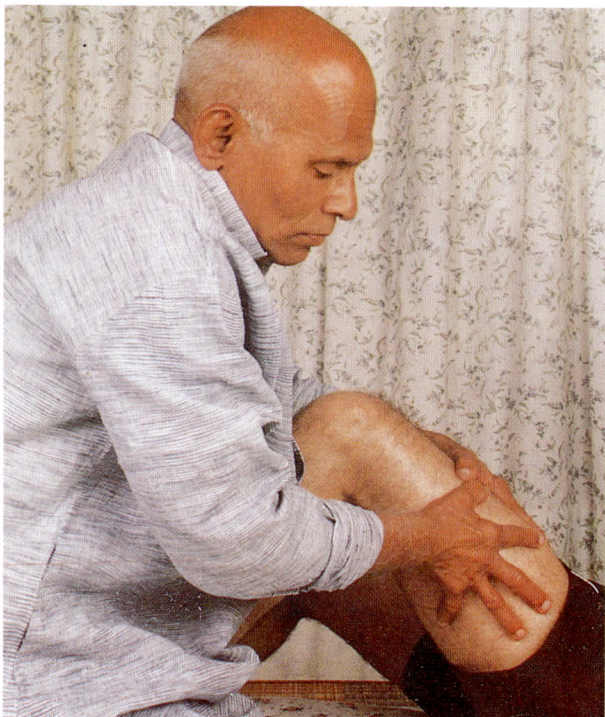

28.   Upper Leg (Kneading)

31.   Lower Leg (Wringing)

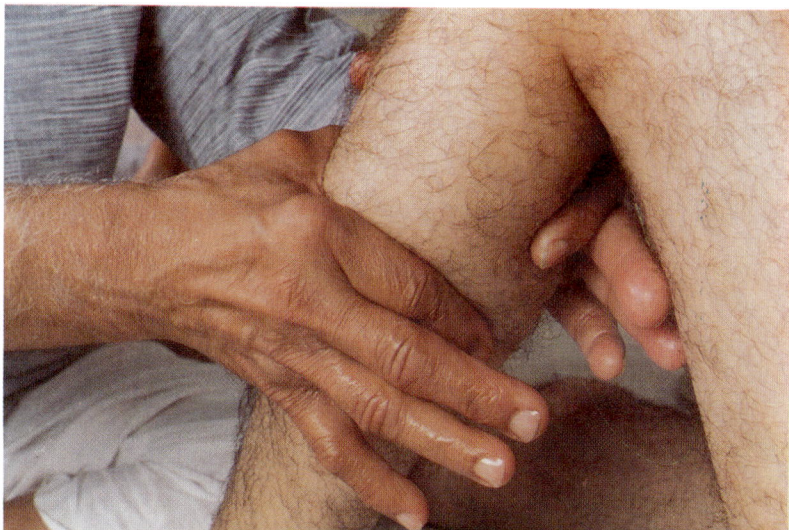

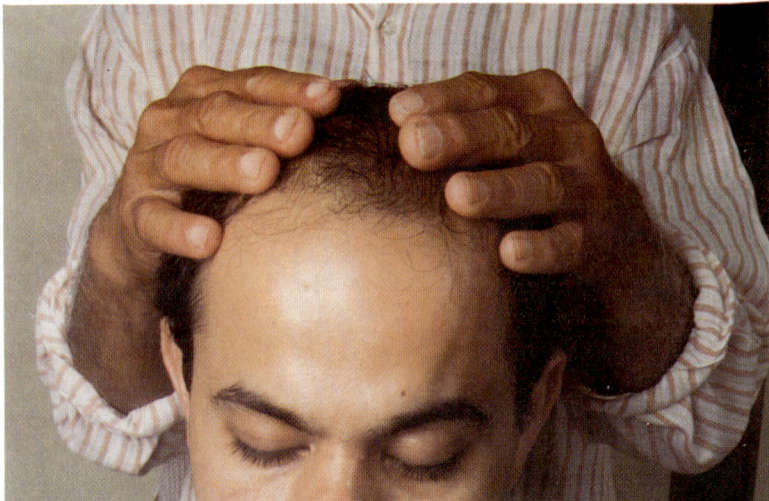

21.   Head Massage (Pounding)

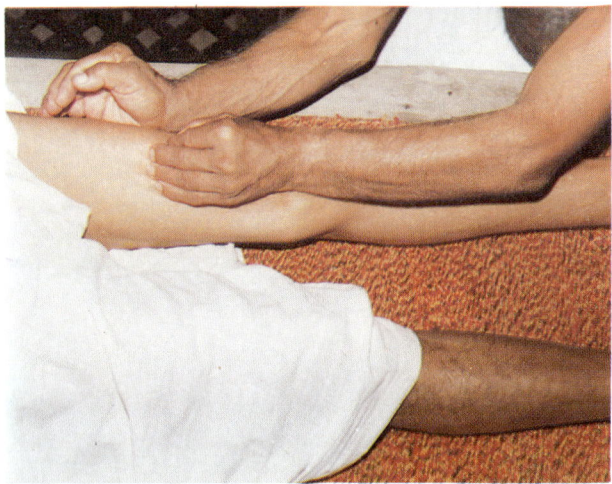

32.   Upper Leg (Clapping)

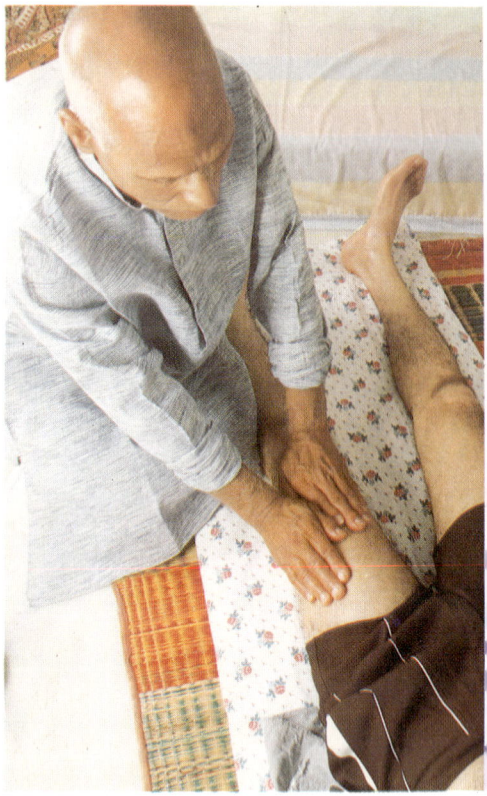

34.   Upper Leg (Pounding)

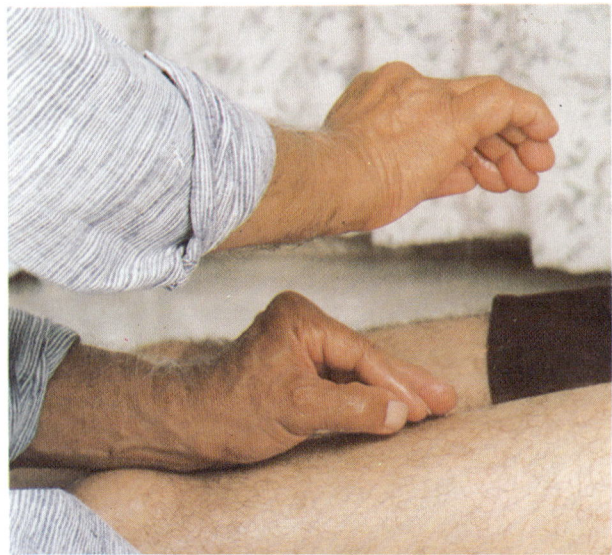

33.   Upper Leg (Clapping)

Massage for beauty starts from the base of the spine (which is fundamental for looking good). Following the spine, massage the arms, forearms, palms, and fingers. Next do the neck and shoulders. Finish with the head and the face. Use milk cream, butter, and special ubatans for skin texture. If skim of milk or pure cream is applied to a girl or boy of any age group, the effect can be seen within two weeks. A week before the massage for beauty actually starts, the diet of the receiver should be fruits, vegetables, nuts, milk, cheese, and cream. This diet should be continued not only during the massage but also for a week after the course is completed.

The massage technique chiefly consists of friction. Not only does it have the power to improve the condition of the skin and the complexion, but also to give lightness and grace to the whole physical form. Use effleurage and kneading as a fundamental part of the treatment. Make the effleurage stroke long and fairly firm; this is designed to mold the figure. In order to remove stiffness or undue firmness of muscles, kneading is necessary. Kneading helps to remove fat and molds the body into graceful curves. Effleurage must be followed by petrissage, which is specially designed to remove imperfections.

The wrists, ankles, fingers, toes and the neck may be given suitable friction. The friction given to the head should be designed to move the scalp and tapotement with the tips of the fingers to stimulate the circulation of blood.

Gentleness of touch is required not only in treating the face but also the whole body. The whole series of movements should constitute one unified effort. The general effect should be soothing, pleasant, and refreshing.

Women generally use a variety of face creams (sometimes very expensive) and talcum powder to enhance their beauty without knowing that massage can do wonders to their appearance in a very natural way. A smooth hand massage on the face can make it glow akin to the moon. Other techniques such as kneading, stroking, vibration, clapping, and so on, may be applied.

Knead the cheeks with the palms. For the head massage use any one of the following oils: Jivanthyadi, Triphaladi, Baladatryadi, Neelibringadi, Kuntalakanthi, Manjishtadi, Eladi, Asabaeladi, Bhringamalakadi, Kumkumwadi, Malathyadi, Brahmi or Nasarshas taila. For explanation of these oils refer to the chapter on oils, pastes and essences.

For the massage of the breasts, women use Yuvathyadi taila because this oil not only enhances the beauty but also restores firmness and youth. For the waist downwards, including the thighs and sex organs of women, Saubhagya Vardhana taila is recommended. At night, before bedtime, massage the face with a mixture of the milk cream with lemon juice and turmeric powder. This will take care of the pimples and acne as well as facial hair.

The duration for a beauty massage may be divided as follows. A total of two hours is required.

1. Spine and back requires 15 minutes and 10 minutes of shavasana (corpse posture).
2. Hands and legs need 30 minutes and 10 minutes of shavasana.
3. Shoulders and neck require 5 minutes with 5 minutes of shavasana.
4. Face and head need 30 minutes with 15 minutes of shavasana.
5. For women, breasts and chest need 10 minutes with 5 minutes of shavasana.

Please note that shavasana is to be done for the prescribed time only after the corresponding area has been massaged. Therefore the total time required is 1 hour and 10 minutes of massage and 40 minutes of shavasana, hence two hours. For women it takes 1 hour 20 minutes of massage and 45 minutes of shavasana (re: step 5).

After the ubatan is removed from the body, a raw milk massage or rose water bath is advised for beauty. In winter, a sun bath after massage is extremely soothing. The hair may be washed with either ritha or shikakai powder, Awala powder, chickpea flour, Multani mitti or yellow clay, yogurt, buttermilk or raw milk. The choice depends on the individual, as per the suitability.

During the beauty massage period, a diet of more milk and fruit juices is essential. Alcohol, tobacco, meat, fish, egg, and so on are strictly prohibited during the course.

AUTO MASSAGE

Auto (Self) Massage. Ordinary massage can be done by oneself. Self massage should never be done in a standing position. Sit and start massaging from the soles of the feet to the head. Different types of massage can be used, though massage of the spine and back cannot be done by oneself.

If an individual obeys the rules of nature, the body can be cleaned thoroughly of all diseases and impurities. The basic testament of a healthy life is a simple, natural diet combined with cleanliness.

Every day the individual should bathe in cold water and walk for about a mile both in the morning and in the evening. Eat well, not to fill one's stomach, but just enough to quench one's hunger and fast once in fortnight. Exercise daily, in the morning or the evening, or both. The exercise schedule should also include shirsasana and pranayama; these are the golden laws of health. All who aspire to a healthy life should follow these guidelines. In case the person practices yogasanas daily then massage is not essential. Oil massage, however, is advised at least once a week so that tissues, muscles, and nerves will be loosened and relaxed.

Daily after a meal, as soon as one washes the hands, rub the eyes with wet palms and move the palms over the face once. This is very good for health.

MASSAGE MOVEMENTS

Massage acts directly on all the three systems, circulatory, nervous and lymphatic. The lymph flows through the ducts, nodes, and passages. It does not flow through capillaries but supplements the blood. The lymph and blood flow side by side. All muscles float in the lymphatic fluid.

The lymph nodes assist in the circulation of blood by draining excess liquid from the blood stream. They also ease the workload of the heart. The lymph provides a direct line of defense to the body. The lymph nodes are activated by the heat produced by friction during massage. By stimulating the lymph flow and generating heat by rubbing oil, massage cleanses and vitalizes the body. That is the main reason why massage rejuvenates the body.

Heat is one of the oldest and most often used forms of treatment. Some examples are hot water bags, heating pads, hydro-collar packs, infra-red generators, and other such heat treatments. Cold packs, massage with wet bath towels or ice cubes, cold bath immersions, and sprays are used for surface cooling. A prime use of heat or cold is for the relief of pain or restoring proper functioning to the affected part.

Use these forms of treatment as well as different movements of the hands and fingers to help in healing various ailments that plague the human race. The following verse has been composed by Vinobaji when I was massaging him. It describes all the important massage movements. I have given the meanings as well as the corresponding techniques.

Mardanam, ardanam, marshanam, sparshanam,
Champanam, kampanam, ladanam, peedanam.
[Kneading, moving, rubbing, touching,
Tapping, shaking, fondling, squeezing.]
The basic movements are described in detail in the ensuing paragraphs.

Effleurage. Effleurage consists of a rhythmic succession of strokes carried out in the direction of the venous and lymphatic flow. While treating the limbs, start stroking at the tips of the extremities and end in the pelvic region, in either the groin or the axilla, in the male and the female respectively. Stroke soothingly to the point of contact, specifically the part undergoing treatment. Generally it is customary to begin massage with effleurage with soothing movements.

Petrissage or Peedanam. Grasp the muscles between the forefinger and the

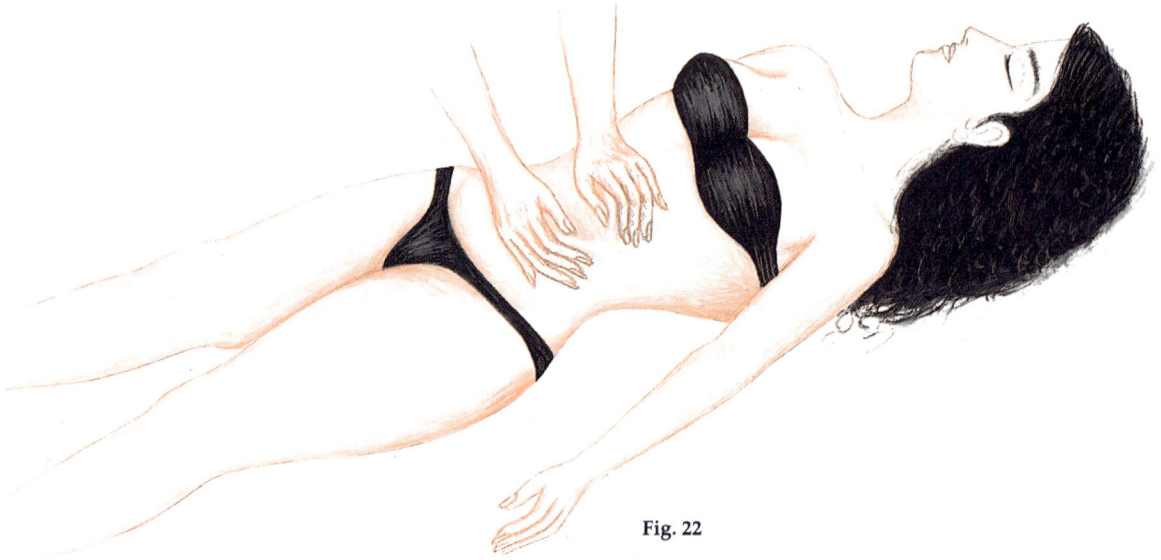

Fig. 22

PETRISSAGE

thumb, lift from the bone and squeeze as shown in Figure 22. Repeat the movement from the head to the toes. This aids in the assimilation of nutrition. Sensitive hands can readily trace the formation of the muscles and feel their response to the treatment. The action of wringing or twisting with regard to the larger muscles is also included in petrissage.

Kneading or Mardanam. Kneading is performed in different ways. Using the fingers, thumbs, and palms of the hands embrace the larger muscles, waxing them into movement and renewing their vitality. For another type of kneading (Photo 28), use your hand to press down on the large surface and move in a circular way, causing the compressing of the soft parts on the harder bone structures. Apply pressure in a wavelike manner. Kneading includes squeezing, grasping, and pinching. Kneading and petrissage help with chorea, varicose veins, recent fractures, inflamed areas, and spastic conditions.

Friction Wringing or Marshanam. Move either with the tips of the fingers or thumbs, the heel of the hand, or the dorsal surface of the two terminal phalanges in small circles. Photos 4 & 31 and Figure 23 illustrate friction wringing. Use this technique to treat patients suffering from lumbago, sciatica, facial palsy, and thickened formations in certain areas of the body. The movement should be in an upward

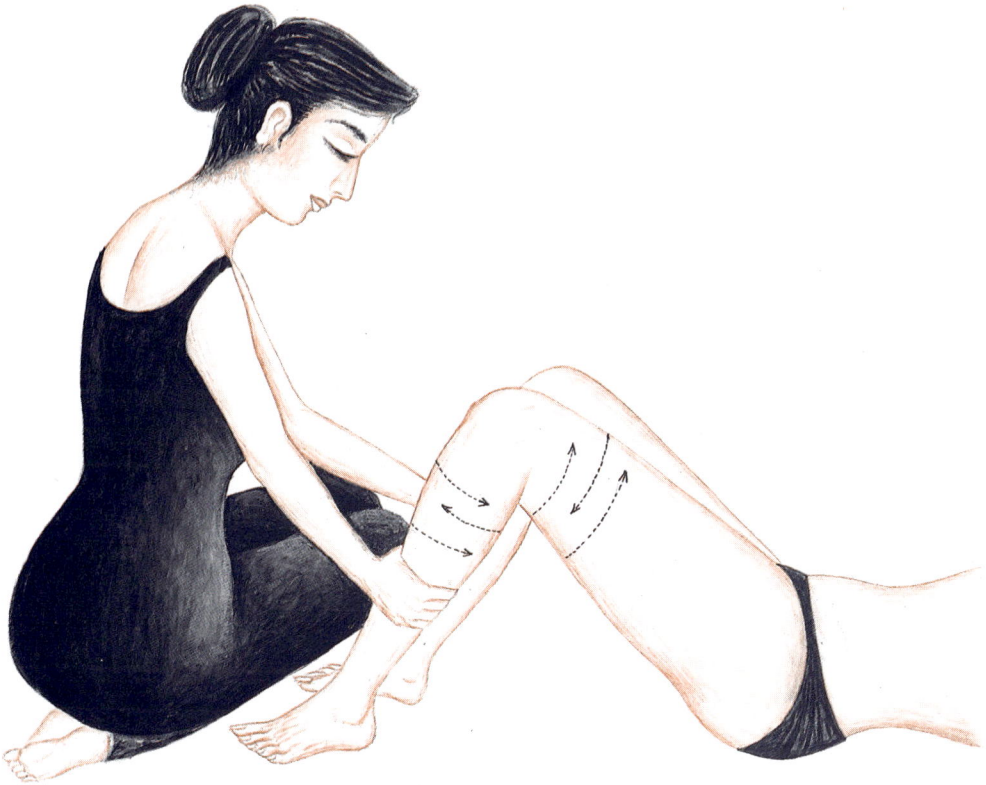

Fig. 23

WRINGING

direction, raising your fingers or thumbs to gain a higher area for a gliding movement, which is similar to a crawling movement. Friction wringing stimulates the smaller tissues.

Tapotement. Six ways to perform this technique include hacking, beating, clapping, pounding, shaking and digital vibrations.

1. Hacking. Use your hands to strike alternately with quick light blows. Do this with the dorsal side of the three inner fingers, the ulnar (inner and larger of the two bones of the forearm) border of the little finger, and the tips of the three middle fingers. Perform this movement from the wrists. Bring the edges of the hands down in short, rapid, alternate strokes, first one hand and then the other, coming into sharp contact with the muscles.

2. Beating (stroking). With your hands lightly closed bring them down from

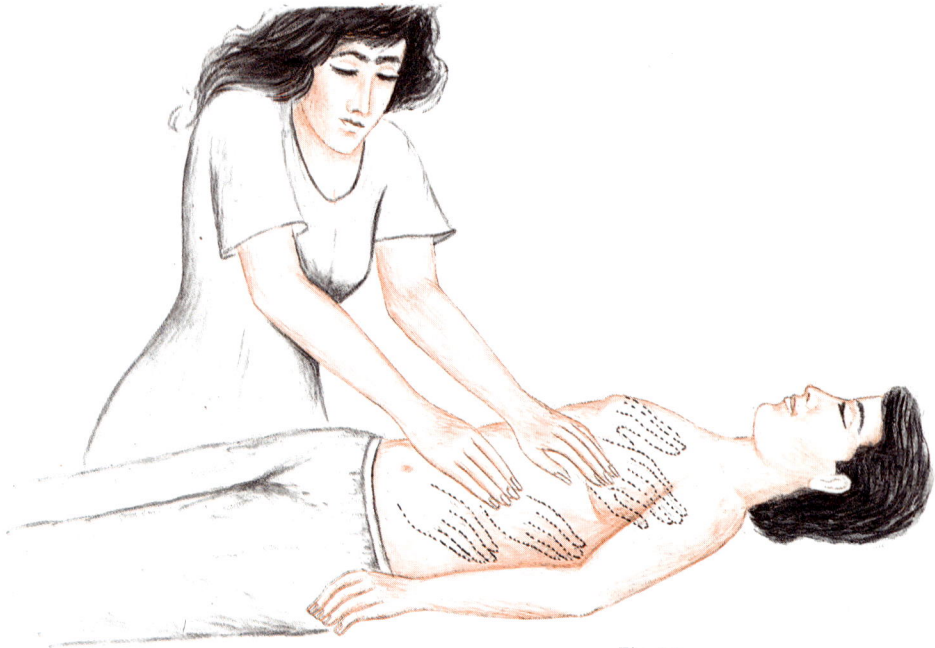

STROKING   Fig. 24

the wrists causing stimulating contact with the tissues that are being treated. Hacking, beating, and drumming are helpful for the large muscles of the loins, such as the lumbar muscles and buttocks. Figure 24 shows stroking and so do Photos 9 and 34.

3. Clapping or Champanam. Clapping is purely a wrist movement, performed with the hands loosely relaxed. Photos 32 and 33 show upper leg clapping.

4. Pounding. Do this with quick movement with the border of loosely closed hands by means of flexion of the hand and extension of the elbow as demonstrated in Photo 36. Use pounding over the liver, buttocks, the fleshy part of the thigh, and on the shoulders, especially in cases of obesity. Beating is a similar movement used for fleshy parts only.

5. Shaking or Kampanam. Hold the limb of concern firmly and shake it in a manner designed to give freedom of action and restore it to its normal condition.

6. Digital Vibrations. In this movement place the middle fingers on the painful parts and vibrate very rapidly, yet lightly. This is helpful in relieving pain in the nerves, as in sciatica. Convey soothing flat-handed vibrations to the affected part

through the surface of the palm. Rest the relaxed hand on the patient. Perform this movement with very rapid contractions and relaxations of the muscles of the forearm.

Stimulating vibrations are good for the sciatica nerve; vibrations are conveyed to the nerve with finger tips, with the fingers remaining stationary, that is, hold fingers together while moving them left and right, sideways, back and forth. Running nerve vibrations are performed by drawing the vibratory fingers down the course of the nerve. General nerve vibrations are conveyed by finger tips along the entire limb. Use digital vibrations in cases of bronchitis, to loosen a much dilated stomach, to dispense flatulence, and to stimulate nerves in cases of facial palsy.

Knead, petrissage, hack, and clap the gluteal region before finishing the back so that you may finish the treatment with friction and stroking down the entire length of the spine. Always knead the gluteal region pressing towards the midline and never separate the gluteal fold. Active or passive, gentle movements may be given to the joints.

Use tapotement to treat liver ailments and to relieve portal congestion which is also associated with the liver. It stimulates the nervous system, helps to break down adhesion, and loosens mucus in bronchitis patients.

Contraindications of this treatment are upper motor nervous lesions, very thin patients, and very painful areas of the body.

OILS, PASTES AND ESSENCES

General Oils. Oil massage offers many benefits. Patting, squeezing, kneading, and striking can be done as part of the massage to the body without oil, but oil softens the skin, lubricates it against friction, disperses heat evenly, provides a glaze, and strengthens resistance to extremes of temperature in the environment. Oil prevents dryness, increases suppleness and durability of the skin and also prevents the effects of premature aging.

For ordinary massage, coconut oil or mustard oil is enough. Generally in Kerala gingelly (sesame) oil is used for massage.

Linseed Oil. Put linseed oil in a green bottle. Linseed oil is better than coconut oil, especially for skin diseases.

Coconut Oil and Lemon Juice. Mix half coconut oil and half lemon juice, then put it in a green bottle.

Mustard Oil. A massage of warm mustard oil cures all sorts of swelling. Massaging it on the stomach cures enlarged spleen.

Olive Oil. In Western countries olive oil is used for cooking and making salads. It is highly praised for being more hot than sesame or mustard oil. It is recommended especially for children, aged, and weak people. It destroys ailments of vata and kapha. It cures swelling, pains, stiffness of muscles, and enhances pigmentation.

Sesame Oil. This oil destroys problems caused by gases, bile, and mucus. Black sesame oil is recommended in Ayurveda to stop greying of hair. It cures gout, arthritis, muscle pain, and swelling. Grey and white sesame oils are medium in quality.

Almond Oil. Use almond oil for revitalizing the brain, nervous system, weakness, old age, and premature aging. This oil is slightly expensive.

Coriander Oil. Coriander oil removes excess body heat.

Pumpkin Seed Oil. Massaging the head with pumpkin seed oil is very good for memory. It also cures insomnia, anxiety and high fever.

Butter and Ghee. Butter is made by fermenting the whole milk into yogurt and then churning it. The butter is heated enough till the water evaporates. Then the ghee is ready which emanates a sweet aroma. The buttermilk, after removing butter, cures vata and kapha and cleans the channels. After food drink a cup of milk and after sex drink a cup of hot spiced milk. Buttermilk is a remedy for piles, assimilation disorders, diarrhea and dysentery and is a treatment for oedema, suppression of urine, loss of appetite, indigestion, anemia etc. Instead of fresh buttermilk nonfat yogurt diluted with equal amount of water and liquefied can be substituted.

Charaka says, ghee the best of all substances is the best to cure both vata and pitta. Cow ghee which is sweet both before and after digestion, is cool, promotes memory, intelligence, the digestive fire, semen and ovum, ojas and fat. It removes toxicity from the system and cures insanity, constipation, and chronic fever. Properly prepared its potency increases a thousand fold and it becomes efficacious in a thousand ways. Aged ghee is used to treat alcoholism, epilepsy, fainting, consumption, insanity, toxic states, fears and pain of vagina, ear or head. The aged ghee is used externally for wound healing and to calm pitta. The ghee of other milk have the qualities of those milk.

Ayurvedic Oils. Each Ayurvedic oil has a medicinal property which helps to heal or relieve the patient/client of many ailments. For general massage, one can use black sesame oil in summer, mustard oil in winter, and coconut oil in spring. Ayurvedic oils can be classified as the following:

1. For Head Massage:

Asana Vilwadi and *Asana Eladi*: Both the oils have same effect. Each promotes comfort of eyes, ears and head and also prevents catarrh.

Bhringamalakadi: Reputed in aches and heat in the head. If applied to the head, it gives comfort to those tired from heavy strain or reading. Gives the eyes coolness, clear vision and natural lustre to its white, black and red parts. Best for the ears and even better for the growth of hair. Important in dental ailments. Those who strain their eyes must use it daily for health and protection. It also improves the voice of musician and gives good sleep.

Triphaladi: Excellent for the head. Specially prescribed for ear and eye ailments. Good for catarrh and tubercular glands.

Chandanadi: Gives coolness and comfort to the head. Good for all ailments due to heat, like fever with burning sensation, alcoholism, confused mind, heat and burning in the stomach and swooning. Very useful in rheumatism, hemothemia and jaundice. Can be used internally, externally and sternutatory. Dosage 5 to 10 ml once or twice daily. For sternutatory 6 to 10 drops.

Balaguluchyadi: Excellent for the head. Good for the body too. Relieves catarrh and allied troubles.

Doorvadi (Coconut oil): Excellent for dandruff and scabies on head.

Vilwapatradi: Reputed in catarrh, dandruff, scabies and other skin diseases on the head.

Nimbadi: Excellent for applying to head in dandruff, scabies and falling hair. Relaxes headache also.

Baladhatryadi: Excellent in heat and ache in the head and eye diseases. Good for any ailment due to vata or pitta above the neck. It can be used externally, internally and sternutatory.

Balaswagandhadi : Good in catarrh, consumption and blood disorders. Reputed for the nourishment and strength of the body. Cures vata diseases, chronic fever, insanity, consumption, cough and other ailments. Can be used for body and head.

Brahmi: Excellent for head and eyes. Gives coolness in the head.

2. For Skin Diseases:

Asana Eladi, Asana Manjishthadi, Durvadi, Vilwapatradi are already mentioned above. Besides these, *Kshara tailam*: Important in ear ailments. Relieves itching, discharge, inflammation, malodor, ache and worms. Best for deafness. Can be dropped or syringed in the ears with bearable warmth. Can be applied in facial and dental ailments.

Gandhaka Tailam: Excellent in itches, scabies in the body.

Gandha Tailam: Good for internal and external use. If applied and massaged, it gives quicker relief to the parts that get sprain, blows or crushing. Reputed for joining fractures and correcting them and for developing limbs. Important in all vata ailments. Dosage 2 to 5 ml twice daily before meals.

3. For Fractures, dislocation and swelling:

Gandha Tailam is mentioned above. Internal dosage strengthens the bones or any deficiency in the bone structure.

Jatyadi : Excellent in wounds. Cloth dipped in it may be laid over the wound; any wound can be cured by purification.

Dhanwantharam Tailam: The effect of this in vata and allied ailments is remarkable. It is inevitable during pregnancy and after delivery. It can be used internally, externally and sternutatory. It is better for pizhichil. It is also prepared in 3, 7, 14, 21, 41 and 101 repetitions. Dosage 5 to 10 ml daily and for sternutatory 5 to 10 drops.

4. For paralysis, polio, rheumatic pains and acute gout:

Ksheeraba Tailam: Most human ailments are due to vata provocation, Tailams control it best, and not better than Ksheeraba. The more it is repeated in preparation, the more effective it is. It can be used internally and externally on head and body, and dhara, pizhichil and vasti. It is good for sternutatory. It is reputed for internal use in facial paralysis, opisthotonos, emprosthotonos, hemiplegia and other nervous dis-orders. Many ailments like vata, cataract, earache, headache, gulma (wind collecting in the belly causing pain, constipation and indigestion and rolling around and pressing upwards and feeling like something solid is the nature of gulma), vaginal disorders and colic are relieved by it. In short, it is the recourse in any ailment connected with vata. In simple vata it is to be applied warm, not so in rheumatism. Dosage 5 to 10 ml once or twice daily. 5 to 10 drops as sternutatory. It is available in 3, 7, 14, 21, 41 and 101 repetitions.

Karpasasthyadi tailam: Good in pounding pain and numbness. Can be applied to the head and body in vata. It is used in hemiplegia and facial paralysis.

Narayana and *Maha Narayana Tailams*: Excellent for vata and vasonita, gulma, colic etc. Useful in chest pain, hemicrania, glands, tubercular glands, stick-jaw, loss of blood and calculus. Maha Narayana tailam is used internally and for sternutatory, it is good for deafness, loss of semen and facial paralysis. It helps women in conceiving. Good in tongue and teeth ailments and insanity. Dosage 5 to 10 ml daily.

Pinda Tailam: Superior in vatasonita and allied burning, swelling, redness, and pounding pain. Good for dhara also.

Prabhanjana vimardana tailam: Important in paraplegia. Very effective if applied externally in pounding pain, numbness and loss of strength. Controls rheumatism and facial paralysis. For quick relief use warm.

Bala and *Mahabala Tailam*: It is good for any vata ailments. It can be judiciously used in excited cough, vomiting, gulma, swooning, chest lesions, consumption and epilepsy. Most effective in facial paralysis and tetanus. It can be used internally and externally or sternutatory, and for shirovasti. Dosage 5 to 10 ml daily.

Vatamardana tailam: Good for any kind of rheumatic pain, sprain and numbness. It is as good as Pinda tailam.

Sahacharadi: Excellent in all vata ailments, especially in cramps. It is also available in 3 and 7 repetitions. Especially in gulma, insanity and vaginal ailments, this shows quick results. Dosage 5 to 10 ml daily.

Rasnadi tailam: Most effective in catarrh, vatasonita and mucus troubles, and also in chronic fever.

Chandanadi tailam is best for acute gout.

5. For mental illness:

Balaswagandhadi and Chandanadi are the oils prescribed for mental diseases. These oils are mentioned above.

Ayurvedic oils mentioned in other chapters:

1. *Tungadrumadi*: It gives coolness to head and eyes.

2. *Tekaraja tailam*: Excellent for applying to the head in cough and asthma. It reduces the heat of the head and sweating.

3. *Mahamasha tailam*: Reputed for internal use and dhara and pizhichil to the limbs with contraction, emaciation and numbness. Effective in hemiplegia, facial paralysis, deafness, locked jaw, sciatica and paralysis on the arms. Dosage 5 to 10 ml daily.

4. *Kachoradi*: Excellent for applying to the body in itches, scabies and all skin afflictions.

5. *Amritadi*: Good for the head in rheumatoid arthritis, sensation of heat on the head, pain and trouble due to pitta provocation. Can be applied on head and body in itches, boils and catarrh afflictions.

6. *Jivantyadi tailam*: Good for sternutatory, in vata, cataract and other ailments. Daily sniffing will benefit optic nerve, retinal atrophy and other disorders and short sight. It also helps any vata or pitta ailments above the neck. For sniffing 2 to 10 drops. Jivantyadi Yamakam is excellent for applying to cracks in feet, palms and lips. Very effective if applied in psoriasis.

7. *Nilibhringadi Tailam*: Reputed for growth of hair; gives comfort to head and

eyes. Good for skin diseases. Same prepared in coconut oil is excellent for internal and external use in spider poison. Dosage 5 to 10 ml daily.

8. *Kumkumadi Tailam*: Excellent for pimples, acne and dark coloring on face. It can be sniffed with Anu tailam.

9. *Anu tailam* : Sniffing is the best treatment for all diseases above neck. It is the best for sniffing to any case. Daily sniffing with it even prevents all diseases of head, eyes, ears, nose and mouth. Sniffing two drops through each nostril in the morning after brushing the teeth and washing hands and feet. By practicing this one can develop broad chest and shoulders, attractive face, sound organ. Our sages proclaim that old age cannot affect them easily.

10. *Malatyadi tailam*: Of proven effect in hair falling due to microbes or other skin ailments on head or body. Best is to start applying after shaving off the hair.

11. *Nasarsas tailam*: Good for head in tonsilitis and nasal polypus (polype).

12. *Yuvatyadi tailam*: This formation is attributed to sage Vatsyayana, and if applied on the breasts regularly, their gradual development, firmness, and shape will not be impaired in old age, according to Vatsyayana.

13. *Saubhagyavardhana Tailam*: Some women suffer from genital diseases, roughness or boils in vagina. Some may have pain also during menstruation. Some may have irregular menstruation. Vaginal application regulates menstruation, smoothens it and satisfies the partners.

6. For retaining youth:

Abhyanga snana (inundation bath) helps to retain one's youth. The person applies oil to one's body from head to toe, without using any particular technique. Daily Abhyanga snana is advised for those who are affected by vata, one of the three components that make up human characteristics. Ksheerabala, Balaguluchyadi, and Karpasasthyadi are recommended. To remove oil after massage when taking a bath, chickpea powder is recommended instead of soap. For patients with pitta, Abhyanga snana is suggested on every alternate day, using Bhringamalakadi and Manjishtadi oils. Manjishtadi oil gives comfort to the head and coolness. It has a pleasant odor, cures catarrh and is good for the eyes. It is good for rheumatoid arthritis. Apply green gram or moong bean powder to remove the oil. Abhyanga snana on every fourth day is advised to kapha patients, using Eladi or Asanavilwadi oil. Eladi is excellent for the head in chronic catarrh. Best for defective teeth, earache, boils and itching, scabies and cold. Chickpea powder may be applied instead of soap. Rinse with clear water.

Solar Energy Oils. The sun's energy makes it possible for any kind of life, plant, animal and human to survive. The properties of solar energy can be harnessed and employed for healing many types of animals. Solar color therapy can be use for healing purposes. It has also been discovered that by focusing on the colors of the prism on to people many diseases can be healed. Natural direct sunshine is fine. Now along with research on many alternative modes of healing color therapy also is being discovered and appreciated. Through the scientific application of color, natural energy is introduced into the body to cleanse, to repair and to heal as light is one of the highest vibrating force of nature.

The seven colors contained in white light are violet, indigo, blue, green, yellow, orange, and red. The first three colors, violet, indigo, and blue fall into the cool part of the spectrum. Green is in the neutral zone, neither hot nor cold. The last three colors, yellow, orange, and red, are in the warm part of the spectrum.

COLORS AND THEIR EFFECTS

1. Violet: Muscles are relaxed by this color. It also acts as an antibiotic, a builder of white corpuscles in the spleen and it depresses the appetite.

2. Indigo: It reduces swelling and pain and firms the skin.

3. Blue: It cures fever, encourages a healing sleep and also stimulates the pineal gland.

4. Green: It has peaceful and calming effects on the body and mind. It cures high blood pressure, hot flashes etc. It raises the vibration of the body over that of disease and heals. It stimulates the pituitary gland and protects from infections.

5. Yellow: It stimulates the nervous system and brain activity. It increases receptivity of knowledge, self-confidence, appetite and enhances liver and gall bladder functions. It also helps to dissolve arthritic deposits.

6. Orange: It invigorates, stimulates and warms the emotions and the glands. It also stimulates confidence, success, proper respiratory functioning, enhances lactation, relieves gas and sluggish digestion, helps brain and brain infections. It decreases menstrual cramp. It is good for those who have paralysis, fears and doubts. Wearing orange scarf around the neck cures thyroid troubles.

7. Red: It stimulates heart-beat and arterial actions and gives energy to the body. It cures anemia, poor blood circulation and cold as it puts a lot of iron and minerals into the blood. It cures kidney, adrenal gland, liver and heart problems. But it is harmful for emotional people.

8. Pink: It cures pelvic problems and helps hip and buttock tenderness. It also stimulates a loving feeling in the heart.

9. Lemon: It cleanses and loosens muscles. It activates the thymus gland and builds bone. It eliminates cold and relieves and soothes muscular tension.

10. Purple: It slows heart-beat and reduces heart pain as it increases venous drainage. It loosens the stiffness, cystic congestion. It also stops excessive menstruation.

Color therapy can be used with three mediums, water, sugar, and oil. The treatment may be internal for which water and sugar are used. Oil is used for external application. Normally red, light blue, blue, and green colored bottles are used for preparing the medium for treatment.

If the patient has fever and other symptoms of heat such as accident injury, use cold color therapy. In case of cold symptoms like cough, throat problem, running nose, paralysis, or arthritis, use warm color therapy. But for infections and enhancing the body's immune system and resistance powers, use green because it is neutral.

Preparation of the medicine. Decide the color of the bottle, wash it and dry it well. Pour the medium you have selected up to three fourths full leaving a quarter for air. Tighten the cork of the bottle. Do not use metal lids. If cork is not available, cover the bottle with a piece of wood. Keep the bottle on a wooden plank in a place where the sun's rays fall on it throughout the day. Before sunset, put the bottle in a wooden cabinet. Take care to see that moonlight does not fall on it. Continue this process for 41 days. When you prepare oil in different bottles at same time, the shadow of the bottles should not fall on each other.

Water should be exposed to the sun's rays for four to six hours in order to derive the benefit of its medicinal properties. Oil and sugar take six weeks or more to prepare. The longer they are kept in the sun the better the results. You can make the medicine during summer months and store it on a window ledge which gets some sunlight. Shake the sugar bottles daily and oil twice a week so that the sun penetrates the entire contents.

Dosage and restrictions. The only restriction is with green color when taken internally. Do not take it within hour of a meal or snack. In case of blue color, it can be taken internally only in extreme cases of hemorrhage, diarrhea or very high fever. The mediums, energized in red or brown colored bottles, are to be taken internally after meals, but no more than a quarter of a cup.

Dosage can be a few grains of sugar several times a day, but should be less than a quarter of a teaspoon. A few drops of oil at a time can be used to massage the affected areas. There are generally no adverse side effects, so do not worry about the dosage. In cases of aggravation, neutralize the effect by taking medicine of the opposite color. You can increase the dosage if necessary.

The results are very quick and effective. At times they are instantaneous, but may take 48 to 72 hours. The cost is virtually nothing. If it works for you, please share this with other friends. Please note that we use brown bottles because they are more easily available than the other warm colors.

Given below are the oils and the colored bottles that they can be prepared with and used for different ailments.

1. Red bottle. The oil prepared in this bottle is warm oil. Generally use it for paralysis, polio, acute gout, and rheumatic aches and pains.

2. Light blue bottle. The oil prepared in this bottle is cool. Use it for ailments of the head.

3. Blue bottle. Though the oil prepared in a blue bottle is also cool, apply it on the chest and back during massage.

4. Green bottle. Oil in a green bottle has antiseptic qualities, hence use it for skin diseases.

Ubatans (Pastes). Ubatans are pastes made from a mixture of ingredients and are used for massaging and also instead of soap during a bath. They have various benefits ranging from cures for illnesses to enhancing beauty.

General purposes. Use one of the four combinations.

1. Soak 2 ounces (50 grams) of lentils in 16 ounces (450 milliliters) of milk and leave it overnight. Make a paste of it by grinding before massaging.

2. Mix well 1 tablespoon of almond oil with 2 ounces (50 ml) of cow's milk cream, add 3 ounces of almond paste and massage.

3. Add almond paste to 1 ounce (25 g) of milk cream.

4. Make a thick paste of 1/4 ounce (5 g) of mustard oil and 2 ounces (50 g) of chickpea flour and one pinch of turmeric powder. Add enough water and apply the paste to the body.

For the Skin

1. Boil and evaporate on a low flame 2 ounces (50 g) of mustard in 9 ounces (1/4 liter) of milk. Dry it in the sun and make a paste of it adding sufficient milk. Apply the paste to the whole body. Allow the paste to remain on the body till it dries. Rub slowly and remove the dried paste and then take a bath.

2. Especially for skin growth. Mix 1/2 ounce (10 g) of mustard oil with 2 ounces (50 g) of chickpea flour along with one pinch of turmeric powder and 1 tablespoonful of fenugreek (methi). Add water and make a paste before applying it on the body.

For Rheumatism

Combine 1/2 ounce (5 g) of olive oil, 1/8 ounce (2 1/2 g) of mustard oil and powders of fenugreek, 1/4 ounce (5 g) of garlic, 2 ounces (50 g) of chickpea and 1 teaspoonful of turmeric. Add enough water to make a paste. Apply this paste to the body.

For Pimples and Boils

Mix 1/4 ounce (5 g) of chiranji paste, 1/4 ounce (5 g) of dried orange skin powder, 1/4 ounce (5 g) of coconut oil, 1/2 teaspoonful of turmeric powder, 1 ounce (25 g) of chickpea flour and a pinch of organic camphor. Mix well while adding enough water to make a paste. Then apply it to the face and body.

After applying the ubatan to the affected parts, relax until the paste starts drying. Rub the pasted area, rolling the peeling paste into a ball. As you remove the remaining paste, dirt will be removed from the skin. The paste provides nourishment to the entire body. With this application, nerves become stronger thus increasing blood circulation as well as energy level in the body. Besides this, it cures disorders of vata, pitta, kapha; it also increases semen, enhancing strength and stamina. Turmeric added to the mixture provides iodine which is absorbed by the skin. The initial application of the paste draws out heat from the body.

For Beauty

Combine 3/4 ounce (15 g) of almond paste, 3/4 ounce (15 g) cashew paste, 3/8 ounce (6 g) of pistachio paste, 3/4 ounce (15 g) milk cream, 1 tablespoon bran oil, 1 tablespoonful rose water, 2 ounces (50 g) red lentils soaked in 3 3/4 ounces (100 g) milk overnight to make the paste. If the paste is too thin, add chickpea flour to it. Apply this to the whole body.

URINE THERAPY MASSAGE

Urine therapy massage is now experiencing a revival. It has been in existence for centuries. In the *Damara Tantra*, an ancient Puranic text, the part entitled Shivambu Kalpa Vidhi discusses ways and means of regenerating one's body with the use of urine. The *Damara Tantra*, which dates back more than 5000 years, records a conversation between Lord Shiva and his wife, Goddess Parvati. More about that later.

The urinary tract is remarkable in construction and design. It has the unrelenting ability to heal and induce vitality into all those who are willing to understand and use it. Its primary function is to create and maintain the salt and water balance and to expel unneeded waste material.

The science of Ayurveda accepts the healing properties of urine. In this form of treatment, the urine of different animals is sometimes used for different internal and external conditions. Now briefly consider the properties of urine and its uses as a medium for massage. Normal urine has the following properties.

1. It is amber colored, clear and sometimes pale fluid which may contain a little mucus.

2. The acid and alkaline properties depend entirely on the person and it has an aromatic odor.

3. It contains 96% water, 2% urea (the product of protein metabolism). It also contains other important minerals like iron, lead, copper, calcium, iodine, magnesium, sodium chloride (common salt), uric acid, acetone, and so on. Vitamins, hormones, and enzymes may also be included.

The use of urine as a therapy affects positively our bodies, minds, and overall health. The antiseptic properties of the fluid are evident in the application of urine on cuts and open wounds. Sometimes urine is used instead of a soap because both urea and ammonia are found in urine.

For massage, old or heated urine may be used. The best urine to be used is the first flow in the morning, about 8 to 10 ounces is most effective. As mentioned earlier, the *Damara Tantra* text explains the process of massage. This passage, taken from the text and translated, tells approximately what Lord Shiva explained to Goddess Parvati.

Now I shall tell you about the process of massage. The aspirant can enjoy the fruits of his practices and meditation utilizing massage with his own urine (V.44). The urine (one's own) should be boiled in an earthen pot until only one quarter of the original remains. Allow it to cool and use this extract for massage (V.48). The aspirant can gain divine powers through this process and he will feel as though he were the king of Gods. He will be free to move where he wishes and will have the strength of ten thousand elephants. He can eat or digest anything (V.49). Never massage urine without first concentrating it to one quarter volume. If this is not adhered to, the aspirant can become dull and prone to disease (V.50). Unboiled urine should never be used for body massage because it is harmful, if used in this way. The aspirant can only gain the benefits of the practice if it is done as directed (V.51). [The verse has been taken from *Amaroli*, which was written by Swami Shankardevananda Saraswati, under the guidance of Swami Satyananda Saraswati.]

The ideas of the West differ from the East in that the West recommends old urine which has matured over 36 hours whereas the East highly supports boiled urine. The East definitely scores because boiling urine to get a quarter of the extract is faster than maturing the urine, a process which in reality requires at least a week and not just 36 hours. The effect of the end products of both the processes, however, is the same. The concentrated urine has more ammonia and a stronger odor, which enables it to enter the body easily.

The process of getting the concentrated fluid ready requires eight to ten ounces of urine. Preserve it in seven bottles over seven days. The urine should be collected everyday, corked, and arranged in the right order for use. Use the older urine first. Make sure that the bottles are cleaned thoroughly and only midstream urine is collected. Shake the bottle well before use.

For the massage, use a bowl, into which half the quantity of urine from the bottle can be poured so that it can be used for one half of the body and the second half for the rest of the body. All movements should be light and in the direction of the heart. From the head downward towards the heart and from the soles of the feet upwards towards the heart. The masseur/masseuse should concentrate on the soles of the feet, hands, head, face, and the back. Use an average time of ten minutes for each part of the body so that the entire massage lasts for an hour and a half to two hours. The patient should not take a bath immediately but wait for at least two hours. The patient should not use soap either.

Due to the heat generated during the massage, one might experience external itching, a rash or even small pimples. The solution is to continue massaging, so that the urine seeps through the cracked skin and heals the wounds. The old or boiled urine can also be used as packs on cuts, inflammation, infections, boils, burns, swelling, wounds, and tumors (cancer). It has been found to be very effective. In case old or boiled urine is not available, fresh urine may also be used.

During one of my visits abroad, a few patients asked me if massage is good for heart patients. I had not treated any heart patient myself, but I did share the experiences of my nephew who used urine therapy about ten years ago. My nephew, an engineer, was working in Dubai in the Middle East. During his stay there he suffered a heart attack and was hospitalized. He was treated in time, soon enough to survive, but the medical doctor advised him to resign and return to India. During a train journey from Kerala to Madras for a tri-monthly check-up, he purchased a copy of *The Water of Life* by J.W. Armstrong on urine therapy. The contents of this book changed the course of his life. My nephew decided to experiment. As the book advised, he stopped all medication and started this new therapy. He continued for three months. When he went for his regular check-up, his doctor told him that all his reports were normal, but insisted that he continue with the prescribed medicines. My nephew then told the doctor about his experiment with urine therapy and how it worked for him. The doctor conducted a thorough check-up again and confirmed that my nephew was fine. Today, after eight years, he is back in Dubai and continues with this magic therapy, massage with urine.

My nephew also treated his mother (my sister) who was a diabetic. He suggested that she discontinue her medication and start auto urine treatment. She once had a carbuncle which was extremely painful. She used urine packs made from three year old urine, keeping it continuously moist with urine. The wound healed within a month.

Some patients I have massaged with urine have had quick results. When I was in Villa Era, Italy, Mr. Giorgio Barabino's sister came to me with severe pain in her shoulders, back, hips, and knees. She was also overweight. I realized that massaging her with any Ayurvedic oil would only increase her weight. I then suggested the idea of massage with her own urine. She agreed and I massaged her for a period of seven days at the end of which her pain had disappeared and she had also lost about four and a half pounds (2 kgs) of weight.

About six years ago, two Italian youths came on bicycles to the ashram from Varanasi, Italy. One of them had a festering, large wound on his leg that had shown no any signs of healing for more than ten days. I asked him if he would allow me to use my medicine and dress the wound. I had stored urine which was three years old which I used to clean the wound. I dressed the wound with a piece of lint dipped in the urine. The next day when I removed the bandage the wound was neither bleeding nor festering. I dressed the wound for another day. Since they had to leave, I suggested that he use fresh auto urine for the wound. He wrote to me from Italy saying that the wound healed very quickly and that the treatment was appreciated.

About four years ago, a lady from Patna came to the ashram. She had a severe condition in her ear that had festered. She had this problem for the past three years and had tried different methods of treatment, but to no avail. Someone suggested my name to her and she came to see me. I told her about urine therapy and she readily agreed because she was willing to try anything. I dressed her ear with three year old urine twice a day for two weeks. When she was leaving, I told her to use fresh auto (her own) urine for dressing her ear. Two years ago she visited the ashram and told me that the problem had not recurred since the magic treatment.

Bhau Phanse, an elderly member of our ashram, developed an allergy which showed no signs of healing despite of a variety of treatments. One day I told him to try auto urine massage, since he had the faith and the experience. He started using fresh auto urine. He too has recovered completely and he continues with the massage even today.

BENEFITS OF AYURVEDIC MASSAGE

Massage helps to increase the production of white blood corpuscles which increases the immunity and resistance power of the body against viruses and diseases. Twelve benefits of Ayurvedic massage are listed.

1. Jarahar (Remover of Old Age). Daily massage to the spine, soles of the feet and head, with almond oil increases virility and semen. The human body is made up of seven components:

Rasa—hormones, fluids and lymph
Rakta—blood
Mamsa—flesh
Medha—tendons of nerves

Asthi—bones, teeth and nails
Majja—marrow
Shukra—semen or ovum

Massage all these seven components for balanced body, which is important for maintaining good health and reducing signs of old age.

2. Shramahar (Remover of Fatigue). Fatigue is caused by physical and mental strain. In turn fatigue affects the muscles and causes tension. Rubbing, patting, and squeezing the muscles gently removes fatigue.

3. Vatahar (Remover of the Humor of Vata). Humor consists of four chief fluids in the body, namely, blood, phlegm, cholera, and melancholy. These determine the physical and mental qualities of a person. Vata causes rheumatism. Daily massage with Maha Narayana taila helps to remove problems caused by vata.

4. Darsanakar (Improves Eyesight). Regular massage improves eyesight and keeps blindness and other diseases of the eyes away. Massage of the feet, especially under the big toe, spine, neck, and head will eliminate eye problems and improve vision.

5. Pushtikar (Strengthener). Rubbing, pressing, kneading, and so on increase and improve the circulation of vital life fluids and strengthen the body on the whole.

6. Ayushkar (Longevity). With regular massage, one can increase the longevity of one's life.

7. Swapnakar (Inducer of Sleep). Ordinarily massage induces sleep but massage of the head and feet with pumpkin seed oil before going to bed can bring deep, peaceful sleep.

8. Twakdhritakar (Skin Strengthener). Massage makes the skin smooth, shining, and strong. Dryness is a sign of the vata element in the body being disturbed. Sometimes dryness is also caused due to anxieties and worries, though people in cold regions develop dry skin due to the chilly weather.

9. Klesha Sahatwa (Tolerance against Diseases). A certain resistance against diseases increases with massage because it stimulates the production of antibodies and strengthens the seven components of the body mentioned in Jarahar.

10. Abhighat Sahatwa (Tolerance against Injuries). A person who receives massage regularly recovers from injuries faster than a person who does not receive massage.

11. Kapha/Vata Nirodhaka (Protector against Phlegm and Wind Ailments). Massage protects the person from all ailments caused by kapha and vata.

12. Mriga Varna Balaprada (Giver of Strength and Color to the Skin). The color, complexion, texture, and strength of the skin improves with massage.

AYURVEDIC MASSAGES OF KERALA

Ayurvedic massage practices typically involve lengthy procedures. The oils used in the three processes/massages may vary depending upon the ailment or physical condition of the patient/client. August, November, and February are the best months for these three treatments.

In Kerala massage is done with Ayurvedic oil at the old age as Kayakalpa.* General massage course is 21 days. Another 21 days rest-cure treatment is also necessary. During the treatment or rest-cure treatment the patient should not do any hard work physically or mentally. The patient can read some spiritual books. He/she should not sleep +during the daytime and his/her head should not sweat. All kinds of movements can be applied according to the condition of the patient. Ayurvedic purgative is also given daily to the patient, if necessary.

For the bath boild water containing some particular Ayurvedic herbs is prepared a night before so that the water should cool enough. The powder of horse gram or chickpea powder is used instead of soap, to remove the oil from the body. Particular Ayurvedic tonic is also prescribed for the patient. After bath tonic is given all the 42 days.

Pizhichil/Squeezing. After having thoroughly examined the patient, the Ayurvedic doctor may prescribe the oil for pizhichil. Heat the prescribed oil slightly. Use old but clean cloth made into a bundle. Ask the patient to lie down in a wooden container which is the size of the average human body (Photo 38). Dip the bundle of cloth into the heated oil, squeeze it slowly. Knead the bundle all over the body of the patient. Do this slowly so that the oil may spread equally with the same amount of heat and then briskly. This technique, of course, is the art of an experienced masseur.

The pizhichil course generally lasts for a period of 14 days. The patient is expected to follow a certain routine for these 14 days to obtain maximum benefit from the treatment. On the first day, massage for one hour. Add 5 minutes daily from the second to the seventh day, on the seventh day the massage lasts an hour and a half. Reduce treatment by five minutes daily from the eighth day onward so that on the fourteenth day the duration is again for one hour.

The masseur/masseuse and the patient/client should take care to see that the patient's head does not sweat. The best time for pizhichil is early in the morning. The patient should not sleep during the day nor should he do any hard work either. As a rule, the patient should not take a bath for the entire duration of the treatment. But in exceptional cases if the patient is to have a bath then it should be under the guidance of the doctor. According to the prescription, the water should be suffi-

---

*About Kayakalpa please refer to Appendix B.

ciently boiled the night before with the necessary herbs. The cooled water can then be used for a bath the next day.

After the 14 days of treatment, the patient is required to undergo a rest-cure period which lasts for two weeks. During the rest-cure period, use the prescribed oil for massage and the indicated boiled water for bath. In order to extract maximum benefit of pizhichil, take special care to see that the patient does not sweat during the treatment or during the rest-cure period.

A wooden shallow tub-like table measuring inside 7 feet long, 2 1/2 feet wide and 6 inches deep is necessary. One end should be higher than the other so that oil applied on the patient should flow. At the lower edge there should be a hole fitted with a tube to collect the oil in a bottle or any other vessel. The head should be covered with a towel dipped in cold water and squeezed so that the massage given with heated oil will not affect the head.

Navarakkizhi (Bundle of Specially Cooked Rice). For this treatment used especially for polio and paralysis, the procedure followed is similar to pizhichil. The difference lies in the making of the kashaya (concoction). To make the rice concoction mix the ingredients listed.

Chop about 3 lbs (1 kg 350 g) of kurunthotti (Sida cordifolia) finely; boil in 3 1/4 gallons (15 liters) of water. Boil until the quantity is reduced to 4 liters (now called kashaya). Take 2 liters from it and add about 2 1/2 pints (1 1/2 liters) of cow's milk and 1 1/3 pints (3/4 liter) Navara rice, a special kind of rice from Navara, generally used for treatment. Cook it well. Then divide the cooked Navara rice into 8 equal parts; tie each part in a small clean cloth. Now you have eight bundles of well-cooked Navara rice. To the remaining 3 1/2 pints (2 liters) of kashaya (boiled water and kurunthotti), add 2 1/2 pints (1 1/2 liters) of cow's milk and boil. Remove from the stove and put the four bundles of rice in it.

Two masseurs/masseuses are required for the massage and treatment, one for the upper body and the other for the lower body. Each one uses two hot bundles in his/her hands and kneads them slowly on the patient's body. The art of this massage lies in the fact that the masseurs simultaneously apply an equal amount of heat and pressure to the patient's body. When they take out four bundles from the kashaya, they put the other four bundles in it. Photo 39 shows four masseurs applying treatment.

This treatment is also given on the table mentioned for pizhichil. While being treated the patient's head should be covered with a wet (cold squeezed) towel.

Dhara/Flow. Dhara means flow. This treatment involves the flow of oil on the body of the patient. Pizhichil and Navarakkizhi are hot massages but dhara is a cold massage. Dhara not only uses oils but also other concoctions. Any one of the following liquids is generally used for the treatment: takram or buttermilk, ksheera or pure cow's milk, tender coconut water, kadi or raw rice washed water, pure fresh water, medicated kashayas, and medicated oils. For the head (Photo 41 — Shirovasti) the following oils can be used: Bhringamalakadi, Manjishtadi, Asanavilwadi, Triphaladi, Chandanadi, Tungadhrumadi and Balaguluchyadi. For the body one can use Pinda taila, Dhanwantara taila, Bala, Ksheerabala, Prabhanjana Vimardhana and Balaswagandhadi. Photo 40 shows this treatment in progress.

Takram for dhara is specially prepared. Put 7 ounces (200 g) of cleaned NAGARMOTHA or MUTHANGA, tied in a piece of cloth, in 2 1/2 pints (1 1/2 liters) of pure milk and add 10 1/2 pints (6 liters) of water and boil till the added water is evaporated. After the milk has cooled down, remove the nagarmotha bundle from it and pour sufficient curd into it. In 5 to 6 hours the milk coagulates and becomes curd. Churn this curd early in the morning and extract the butter. The buttermilk can then be used for dhara. While churning the curd, use filtered MUTHANGA KASHAYA instead of cold water. So from 2 1/2 pints (1 1/2 liters) of milk, 5 pints (3 liters) of buttermilk will be ready for dhara.

Dhara with ksheera is made with freshly extracted cow's milk. Ayurvedic medicines such as chandan or sandalwood paste, camphor, and panchagandha are generally added. These Ayurvedic medicines should be made into a fine paste before adding them to the milk. For dhara, a droni or wooden boat-shaped vessel fitted on a table, made of teak wood or rosewood, is required. The droni should be about 7 ft long, 2 1/2 ft wide, and 10 inches deep. One end is usually a little higher than the other. At the lower end is a hole fitted with a tube by which the liquid used for dhara can be collected in a bottle or vessel. The patient lies in the droni, keeping his head at the higher end. The liquid collected in the bottle or in a vessel can be used twice or thrice during the day (on the same patient). The oil should flow towards the legs at the lower end so it can be collected in the pit of the wooden vessel.

Use a kindi (pot) (Figure 25) made of gold or silver for dhara. You may also use an earthen kindi if a gold or silver one is not available. Make a small hole at the bottom of the desired pot and fit into the hole a suitable yarn wick. Hang the pot over the wooden vessel in which the patient is lying. Pour the prescribed liquid, oil, takram or ksheera in the pot. Allow the liquid to trickle onto the body of the patient. Start the treatment at the head and move down to the feet. For dhara, one well-experienced masseur/masseuse and two assistants are required to work under the guidance of an expert Ayurvedic doctor. The masseur/masseuse and his/her assistants must take care of the patient's daily routine during the course of the treatment. The duration of the treatment is similar to Pizhichil and Navarakkizhi.

The treatment lasts for one hour. Pour 5 1/2 pints (3 liters) of liquid over the patient in 20 or 25 minutes. Then reuse the same liquid, collected in the pit of the wooden vessel, until the treatment of the day is completed. Apart from the already mentioned requirements, the treatment needs more equipment: 3 stools, oil for the head, oil for the body, chickpea or moong or green gram powder in place of soap, and the necessary pieces of cloth.

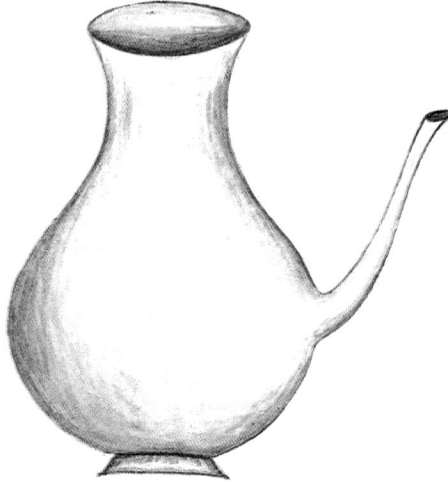

Fig. 25

KINDI (EWER OR PITCHER)

Dhara can be given to specific parts of the body such as only the head, any particular limb, only the eyes, or the whole body.

DOING MASSAGE WITH LEGS

In Kerala, some expert masseurs and masseuses massage patients using their legs. A long, smooth, and strong rope is tied to the ceiling (see Photos 42-44). The masseur/masseuse holds the lower end of the rope while he/she uses his/her legs to massage the patient who is lying down on a mat just below the rope. A plate with enough oil is kept handy. The masseur/masseuse uses the soles of his/her feet similar to the way hands can be used. If the patient is strong enough the masseur/masseuse can use the soles of both feet for the massage on the back, waist, and buttocks of the patient.

III HEALING THROGH MASSAGE

CASE STUDY SUMMARIES

In the past 23 years, Govindanji has cured patients suffering from a variety of ailments through the wonderful art of massage. Here are a few examples.

1. Shri Shivaji Bhave, the younger brother of Acharya Vinoba Bhave, had an accident which caused him to suffer from multiple fractures on his right thigh. After the plaster cast was removed he was unable to walk or do any of the exercises prescribed by the doctors. He then underwent massage with medicated Ayurvedic oils for a month and gradually he was able to walk without the help of a walking stick.

2. Shri Babulal Mittal of Agra, who was a member of the ashram, had a severe paralytic stroke. Govindanji massaged him regularly with medicated Ayurvedic oils in conjunction with taking Ayurvedic medicines internally, which were prescribed by a doctor. After a few months of this treatment, Babulalji was able to walk again, as before.

3. A gentleman from Padaso, Italy, came to Govindanji complaining of insomnia. During the massage session, the gentleman started snoring.

4. A 16 year old girl from Biella, Italy, complained about irregular menstrual cycles and also of irregular bust growth. She underwent massage for a period of 15 days, after which her menstrual cycle became regular and her bust size also increased.

5. In Borgoseria, Italy, a 25 year old woman had a fall in the snow while skiing. In the hospital her left leg was put in a plaster cast. After the plaster was removed, she found that she was unable to stretch her leg. The doctors who were treating her suggested exercises, but they had no effect. The next alternative was surgery. She immediately got in touch with Govindanji. He massaged her leg with a special oil, both in the morning and in the evening for three days. She had been unable to walk without the help of a walking stick. After several weeks of continued treatment, she was able to start her Karate lessons without any problem.

6. A pregnant woman, aged 40, came to see Govindanji when he was in Turin, Italy. She told him that she had several miscarriages and that she was very keen on having this baby. Govindanji told her that he was not a doctor, but he massaged her while he was in Turin. His student continued after he left. Several months later Govindanji received a letter from the student saying that the woman had a normal

delivery without the help of a doctor and that both the mother and the child were in good health.

HEALING THROUGH MASSAGE

This section covers prevention and treatment. One proverb states that prevention is better than cure. As a preventive against illness, daily auto massage is very beneficial. It is important to remember in massage that the direction of the strokes should be towards the heart. The prevention aspect has already been explained in the previous chapters. In this chapter we shall talk about the different techniques used to cure or relieve certain ailments.

General Rules

Lower Body. In order to treat the lower limbs and muscles, friction is necessary. Place the tips of the fingers or thumbs on the affected part. Then move the tissues beneath the surface with circular movements, taking care to maintain the pressure and to avoid the error of allowing the fingers or thumbs to glide over the surface. Keep moving your hands in small circles and repeat in an upward direction, raising the fingers and the thumbs to reach a higher area. Though deep pressure is required on the upper tissues, press on those beneath. Do not apply undue force. This movement is of special value on the obstacles which cannot be kneaded. Apply it to the spine, tendons, and joints. In treating the spine give friction in close proximity to each of the joints, dealing with both sides with careful circular movements.

Upper Body. Neck massage should be in circular motions towards the jaw bone using the thumbs together or in turn while the fingers lightly grasp the neck. Stiffness of the neck can be cured by this movement which goes mainly to the back and sides of the neck. Friction, petrissage, and effleurage, all very gentle movements, may be given to the face. Start with light stroking to relax the obstacles. The friction on the head should be in small circles, so that the scalp on the bone is massaged, which helps circulation.

Diseases of the Nerves

1. Sciatica. Neuralgia of the large nerve of the thigh is known as sciatica. Treatment starts with effleurage in long soothing strokes down the full lengths of the nerve. Friction may also be used. A major part of the treatment is given to the buttock where the head of the curve is set. Deep pressure may be applied, as much as the patients can endure, avoiding the inflamed nerve itself. Rubbing at the points of pain mainly the hip bones, waist, thighs, and ankles is required. Sunbathing helps this situation. Effleurage is definitely soothing and should follow all friction treatment. Ask the patient/client first to place one hand on the kneecap and the other under the joint, raising the leg as far as possible without causing great pain, thereby stretching the nerve. Then have the patient/client bend his/her knee and draw the

whole limb back to the abdomen. Now use effleurage not only for the buttock but the whole length of the leg.

2. Rheumatism. Give general massage paying special attention to any part that threatens to cause pain. Ask the patient/client to breathe deeply and do other physical exercises on a regular basis. Then deal with the area affected by rheumatic conditions, particularly with unhealthy and painful muscles. All the leading massage movements may be applied. Petrissage combined with kneading, deep friction, and beating produces good results. The aim is to reduce inflammation and soften the fibrous tissues.

3. Arthritis. The dreaded word indicates the inflammation of joints which as in rheumatoid arthritis or as in traumatic arthritis, are affected alike. For this ailment, start with fomentation for 3 minutes with warm water, followed by a cold pack for 1 minute and again with warm water fomentation for 3 minutes. Then massage with Sahacharadi, Mahanarayana or Prabhanjana Vimardana taila. After massaging, apply a day pack on the affected area for about 3/4 of an hour. This treatment should be continued for 41 days.

Rheumatoid arthritic joints often appear swollen and red and the pain sometimes increases whenever that joint encounters movement. In such a case, do not massage on the actual joints, but apply effleurage and kneading above the affected parts. Massage can assist greatly and can correct or improve ailments such as constipation and circulation.

4. Rheumatic Pain. The pain is due to excess alkaline in the body. So massaging in the direction of the heart will give relief. Pressure should be given around the affected joints. Kneading, friction and vibration can be applied during massage. Steam fomentation, sweating and massage, the three combined, can work miracles.

5. Polio. Children sometimes contract this disease after a bout of typhoid. In the early stages of disease, massage with cod liver oil gives the best result. Massage techniques should include kneading of the muscles, petrissage, effleurage, wringing, clapping, and vibration. Back massage is also essential. Massage the patient twice a day for 30 minutes each time. Exercise the affected parts up to a point, until the patient does the exercise independently. After the exercise the patient should lie in Shavasana for 10 to 15 minutes. Use fish oil or Mahanarayana oil.

6. Paralysis. Paralysis is often the outcome of shock, disease, or injury. Loss of motor power and sensation are among the main symptoms. The body may be paralyzed vertically from head to foot, or on one side only. The side of the brain which is affected is opposite to the side which is paralyzed. The usual massage movements may be given. Apply the medicated Ayurvedic oil prescribed by a doctor. Effleurage, petrissage with kneading, and tapotement, are especially helpful to the unaffected side of the body. Local paralysis may affect a hand or a leg or one side of the face

or the other parts of the body. General massage with medicated oil giving effleurage to the paralyzed limbs has remarkable virtue.

Massage with oil prepared in a red bottle or any one of the oils such as Mahanarayana taila, Pinda taila, Prabhanjana Vimardana, Kuzhampu, and Ksheerabala. Kneading, petrissage, wringing, stroking, friction and vibration may be applied during massage. Exercise is vital to the affected joints. Pizhichil or Navarakkizhi also may be given as a treatment.

7. Leprosy. The patient can continue with other courses of treatment. For massage, the affected parts are first smoothened with pure melted wax (100°F-120°F or 38°C-49°C). Use neem oil, Mahamasha taila or Kachoradi taila for massaging the affected parts.

8. Reducing nervous tension. Sensory nerves convey impulses or messages to the brain, while motor nerves relay messages from the brain. The central nervous system is composed of the brain, the spinal cord, and the nerves. The spinal nerves pass between two vertebrae and are distributed all over the body to the joints, muscles, and the skin. Use gentle effleurage along the full lengths of the spine, from the lumbar muscles to the nape of the neck for a remarkable effect.

The movements should be slow and should be repeated again in a soothing rhythm. In cases of nervousness, a sympathetic hand may smooth and relax the patient. The massage may be able to ease disturbing conditions such as nervous debility and hysteria. Massage gives the desired result and also benefits the physical condition of the patient.

9. Madness. For this ailment, use a combination of massage techniques along with other prescribed courses of treatment. Massage of the head, neck, and back, using oils such as Bhringamalakadi, Manjishtadi, Aliquot, Amrutadi, Chandanadi, Tekaraja or oil prescribed in a light blue bottle. Treat twice a day, once early in the morning and once at night before bedtime. In summer, use cold massage for the neck and back for good results. Use the techniques of petrissage, stroking, clapping, and vibration for about 30 minutes.

10. High Blood Pressure. First and foremost, the patient should abstain from alcohol and smoking. A well-balanced and controlled diet, along with other courses of treatment is essential. Give smooth massage for the head and feet to relieve pressure on the arteries. To help purify the blood, the patient should drink more water than usual. Use smooth massage, smooth clapping, and slight vibration techniques for not more than 15 minutes. Using Shavasana for 15 minutes after massage aids in curing the patient. Uninterrupted lymph flow reduces blood pressure. Massage is helpful for a patient with high blood pressure. It also relieves aches and tensions and promotes deeper, more natural breathing.

Diseases of the Abdomen

1. Constipation. Many maladies have been traced to poisonous matter in the

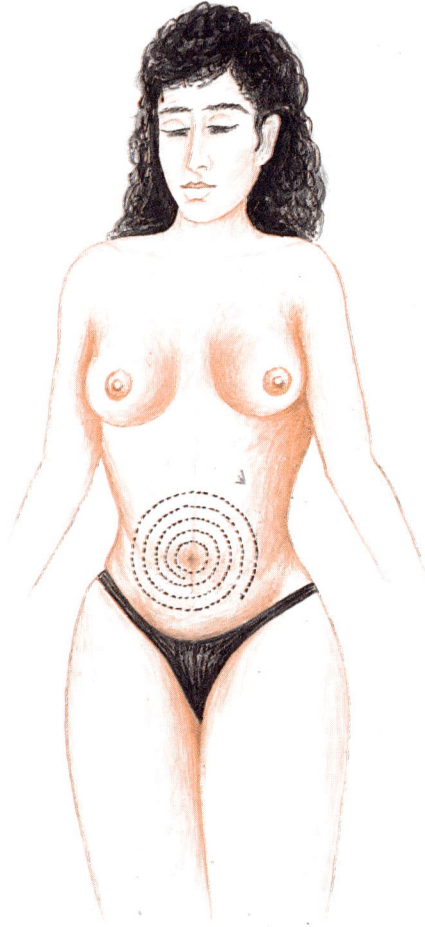

MASSAGE FOR CONSTIPATION

Fig. 26

bowels. Constipation is a frustrating affliction with the tiresome need of resorting to purgatives. To stimulate the action of the bowels by natural means, massage has proved to be a most effective aid. When treating the abdomen, the bladder should be empty. Be sure the patient/client has no inflammation or ulcers. Abdominal massage is not advisable during pregnancy.

During abdominal massage (Figure 26) ask the patient to raise his/her knees. Use effleurage and gentle kneading on the abdomen for good results, particularly in cases of convalescence. Complete relaxation of the abdominal muscles is essential. Ask the patient to sit on the right side of the masseur so that he can give gentle effleurage in a clockwise direction over the entire abdominal area. Start with light kneading, gradually making the kneading firmer and deeper. Repeat the same procedure from the downward pressure in small circles. Treat one limited area after another so that the underlying tissues will feel the impact. Deep effleurage should follow the above procedure.

Friction should be applied over the whole inner area of the abdomen commencing from the center and working on the small intestine. Give deep kneading over the entire abdominal area. Sometimes just gentle massage will bring the desired effect. Stroking with the finger tips will also help to ensure beneficial contractions.

2. Obesity. Food free from fat and sweets, yogasanas and proper exercise are very essential for the obese patient/client. Cold massage or massage with one's own urine brings better results. Apply kneading, wringing, tapping, and clapping.

3. Slimness. A balanced diet, yogasana, exercise, and life free from mental worries and tensions is must for the underweight patient. Oil massage will then be very effective. Use kneading, wringing, stroking, clapping, and vibration techniques.

4. Sleeplessness. This ailment depends upon the stomach. When one gets too little sleep, nerves become weak. Another cause of sleeplessness is mental tension. A balanced diet coupled with exercise is essential. A good way to exercise is to walk for a distance of one mile, twice a day. Listening to any spiritual discourses or positive affirmations helps one to get good, sound sleep. Soothing soft music also helps. Massaging the whole body before going to bed is advisable. Take special care during the head and back massage. Cold massage for the head is very good. Use smooth movements such as tapping, clapping, and slight vibration techniques. Hot massage for the soles of the feet is also important. The patient may soak the legs (from the sole to the knee) in hot water (120°F) for 10 to 15 minutes. Make sure that the temperature of the water is constant. After the prescribed time, wipe the legs dry and massage the soles of the feet using either Ksheerabala, Prabhanjana Vimardana taila, or Pinda taila.

5. Piles and Prostate. Patients with piles or prostate problem can deal with it by putting oil on the tip of a finger and inserting it into the anal opening and turning it 5 to 6 times.

General Injuries

1. Inflammation. The medical treatment of a dislocation or a fracture may be performed by a surgeon. Massage can be given later. Use effleurage for the injured limb, paying special attention to the areas above and below the injury. At a later stage, deeper effleurage, combined with petrissage, such as kneading, will definitely help in restoring the normal condition of the muscles. Effleurage in the form of cautious stroking aids in easing pain and reducing inflammation.

2. Fractures. (1) Wind a long piece of cloth that has been dipped in Dhanwantara taila or Gandha taila around the affected portion. Then place enough cotton over it to cover the fracture supported by two bamboo sleeves; tie the bandage. Take care to see that the bamboo strips do not touch the skin and that the affected part cannot move until the fracture heals completely. Every third day massage for 15 minutes using Dhanwantara taila. The bandage should be tied back over the fracture as soon as treatment is finished. Continue this treatment for 15 or 21 days as the case may be. Smooth massage with Dhanwantara taila may be given for 15 minutes twice a day, morning and evening. After a week, petrissage and smooth vibration can be applied along with simple exercises.

(2) Compound Fracture. After aligning the broken bones, bandage the affected portion as mentioned above. If there is a wound, then the bandage should not be removed until the wound has healed. Vranaropana taila is generally applied for healing a wound. After 15 or 21 days, treatment with Dhanwantara taila should be given every fourth day. Massage with Dhanwantara taila is advisable for another 2 to 3 weeks. Simple exercise to the affected part can be given.

AYURVEDIC HERBS AND FOOD COMBINATIONS

What effects do tridoshas have on human beings? Everyone should be aware of the influence doshas have on our daily diet. Food has been classified according to the doshas. These doshas can determine the nature, personality, mental make-up, and physical features of a person.

In Ayurveda, yoga refers to the right usage and combinations of herbs. Yogic usage of herbs implies a harmonious application of the potencies of the herbs. Healing is always a process of unification. Man as a microcosm contains within himself all the elemental, mineral, vegetable, and animal kingdoms. Within the plant is the potential of a human being, and conversely, within the human being is the underlying energy structure of the plant. For example, our nervous system is a tree whose plant essence is human. The plant kingdom exists to bring feeling into the manifestation of life. Consciousness in plants is a primal level of unity. Therefore it is more psychic and telepathic.

The earth inhales and exhales stellar and cosmic forces, the absorbed essence of which grows and manifests as life. These forces are not on the material plane, but include subtle energies of an occult or spiritual nature. Plants transmit the vital emotional impulses and the cosmic energies emanated by plants nourish, sustain, and give growth and energy to our bodies or astral bodies.

Prakriti (nature) consists of three basic qualities (gunas), satwa, rajas and tamas. The principles of light, perception, intelligence, and harmony are the qualities of satwa. The principles of energy, activity, emotion, and turbulence are the qualities of rajas. The characteristics of tamas are inertia, darkness, dullness, and resistance.

Ayurvedic Herbs

Ayurveda classifies herbs into three gunas, each with qualities for developing certain psychological responses. Satwik herbs promote the development of the mind and enhance its clarity. Rajasik herbs contain energy which comes from fire. Tamasik herbs contain inertia which comes from the earth.

These three gunas have a corresponding effect on the plant kingdom, which in turn affects the three doshas. The roots of trees correspond to the earth and water, hence kapha. Flowers correspond to fire, therefore pitta. Leaves and fruits correspond to the ether, thus vata.

Psychological factors have the power to overcome diseases and their adverse effects. Ayurveda is a science which allows us to make use of herbs to help counteract mental and emotional problems. In Ayurveda, treatment is given to the individual according to the constitution governed by the predominant dosha. For example, dry and heat producing herbs are used for kapha which is cold and moist. Heat producing and moist herbs are for vata which is cold and dry. Cooling and dry herbs are for pitta which is hot and moist. The constitution of the individual represents vulnerability to diseases. For example, people with kapha qualities are prone to diseases like cold and congestion. Disease conditions of a different nature than those of individuals who are relatively easy to treat. Those of the same nature are more difficult to treat since the nature of the individual reinforces the nature of the disease.

Herbal medicines that reduce kapha in a person are predominantly bitter, astringent, and pungent in taste. Treat pitta with pungent herbs like ginger and bitter tonics. Use pungent herbs to treat obstructed vata. Ayurvedic treatment to reduce vata contains rock salt.

What effect does each one have on the human constitution?

Sweet. Sweet food promotes the growth of all the body tissues, aids longevity, ensures smooth functioning of the five sense organs of the body and gives strength to the body. It alleviates pitta, vata, and effects of poison. Sweet food relieves thirst and a sense of burning. It promotes the healthy growth of skin and hair. It is good for the voice, induces energy, and is nourishing and revitalizing. Sweet food helps to create firmness and it removes weakness. It refreshes the nose, throat, lips and tongue. It is wet, cooling, strong, and heavy. But an excess of sweet food has many adverse effects: obesity, laziness, excessive sleep, a heavy feeling about oneself, loss of appetite, difficulty in breathing, cough, retention of urine, fever, cold, goiter, and swelling of lymph glands, legs and neck. An accumulation of sugar in the bladder and blood vessels increases kapha-related diseases. Limit your consumption of sugar.

Sour. Sour substances add taste to the food, enkindle the digestive fire, make the mind alert, give firmness to the sense organs and the heart, increase strength, dispel intestinal gases, and promote saliva which helps swallowing and digestion of food. Sour produces heat and is wet and heavy. Excess sour food makes the teeth sensitive, and increases thirst and the frequent blinking of eyelids. Sour food lique-fies kapha and aggravates pitta. With its heat producing property, it promotes the maturation and suppuration of sores, wounds, burns, fractures and other injuries. It causes a burning sensation in the throat, chest, and heart. Sour foods are harder to find than sweet foods. Berries, lemon, lime, raspberries, and rose-hips are sour.

Salty. Salty food promotes digestion and enkindles the digestive fire. It is a sharp, corrosive fluid that acts as a sedative and a laxative. Salty food alleviates vata, relieves stiffness, causes contractions of muscles, and induces softness. It promotes salivation, liquefies kapha, and cleanses the blood vessels. Salty food is moderately heavy and heat producing. An excess of salty food aggravates pitta, causes stagnation of blood, increases thirst, fainting, and sensation of burning in the throat and ab-domen. It also aggravates infectious skin conditions, causes symptoms of poisoning, ruptures, and tumors. Such food induces the falling out of teeth and decreases virility. Salty food promotes hyperacidity, gout, and other pitta diseases.

Pungent. Pungent food cleanses the mouth, enkindles the digestive fire, puri-fies food, promotes nasal secretion, causes tears, and gives clarity to the sense organs. It helps to cure intestinal diseases, obesity, abdominal swelling, and gets rid of excessive liquid in the body. It discharges oily, sweaty and sticky waste products. It kills worms, corrodes muscle tissue, helps to remove blood clots, facilitates proper circulation of blood, and alleviates kapha. An excessive amount of pungent food weakens virility. Because of its potency it causes weariness, languor, emaciation, fainting, dizziness, and delusions. It generates a burning sensation in the throat as well as in the body. It diminishes strength and increases thirst. Pungent food is light, strong, dry, and heat producing. Spicy and aromatic herbs are included in this category. The herbs are angelica, asafoetida, cayenne, ginger, basil, bayberry, bay leaves, black pepper, camphor, cardamom, horse radish, mustard, cumin, eucalyptus, garlic, cinnamon, cloves, coriander, onion, peppermint, prickly ash, and rose-mary.

Bitter. Bitter food detoxifies, creates tightness of the skin and muscles, en-kindles the digestive fire, and promotes the digestion of toxins. It purifies lactation, melts accumulated fat, and helps to remove toxins from fat, sweat, urine, excreta, pitta, and kapha. It is strong, cool, dry, and light. Excess usage of bitter food causes a wasting away of all the tissues and elements in the body. It produces roughness of the skin, takes away strength, and causes emaciation, weariness, delusions, dizziness, dryness of the mouth, and other diseases of vata. The herbs in this category are bayberry, blessed thistle, blue flage, dandelion, golden seals, peruvian bark, rhu-barb, tansy, yarrow, and yellow dock.

Astringent. This acts as a sedative, arrests diarrhea, and aids in healing aching joints and open wounds. It acts as a drying, firming and contracting agent. Astrin-gent food alleviates kapha and pitta and helps in the clotting of blood, especially in open wounds. It promotes the absorption of bodily fluids. Too much astringent food causes dryness in the mouth, produces pain in the chest near the heart, causes constipation and weakness of the voice, obstructs circulation of blood, and darkens the skin. It also weakens vitality, causes premature aging, and retention of gases and urine. Astringent food can also cause emaciation, increase thirst, and cause stiffness of muscles. Excess astringent food causes diseases of vata like paralysis, spasms, and convulsions. The herbs in this category are lotus, mullein, plantains, pomegranate, raspberry, sumac, uva ursi, white pond lily, and white oak bark.

Combination of tastes. Combinations of certain foods and herbs have a variety of effects on the human body. Sweet and astringent herbs are good for kapha; they include bayberry and cinnamon. Bitter and astringent herbs such as golden seal and uva ursi are good for pitta. The food we eat deals with the grosser part of nutrition while herbs give subtle nutrition and stimulation to the deeper tissues and organs in the body.

Tastes and Emotions. As mentioned earlier, the prakriti of the gunas and doshas has a great part to play in determining the constitution of an individual human being. Here are the different tastes and the kinds of emotions associated with them:

1. Bitter — grief; astringent — fear; both aggravate vata.
2. Sour — envy; pungent — anger; both aggravate pitta.
3. Sweet — desire; salty — greed; both aggravate kapha.

Food Combinations

Certain food combination qualities disturb the doshas as well as the gunas which leads to illness and disease. Avoid certain combinations to maintain good health.

1. Raw and cooked food should not be mixed at the same meal, unless the amount of one is much less compared to the other. For example, a little raw chutney or a paste made of raw ingredients is okay to serve in a small quantity.

2. Fish and milk should not be combined.

3. Equal amounts of honey and ghee should not be combined.

4. Excess of any quality of food is forbidden. Alcohol, yogurt and honey are foods that produce heat. Therefore other heat producing foods should not be combined with them.

5. You may change the rules in combining food in order to provide an anti-dote. For example, the consumption of milk and radish, together, is prohibited because milk is cold and radish produces heat. But when they are consumed to-gether in the right proportion they provide an antidote that helps digestion.

Charaka said that even food which is the giver of life to human beings, if taken in an improper manner, destroys life. But if taken in the proper proportion and combination it acts as an elixir. I have enlisted some of the rules which will help you to lead a balanced life.

1.   Eat cooked food to stimulate digestion.

2.   Eat unctuous food, which excites the digestive fire and nourishes the body.

3.   Eat well-combined food in the proper measure and be sure to have a balanced interval between two meals. This helps in the proper digestion of food.

4.   Eat in a congenial, quiet place so that your mind is not disturbed or depressed.

5.   Eat your food at a moderate pace so that the gait of the food, as it moves through the digestive tract, will be balanced.

6.   Eat with concentration and pay attention to what you are eating. Prefer-ably, remain silent during your meal so that your meal gets your undivided attention. Focus on your constitution and avoid those foods which may cause harm.

7.   Do not eat if you are not hungry.

8.   If possible, sit facing the East when you have a meal.

9.   Say a small prayer of thanks before you start eating.

10.   Take a stroll of about a 100 steps after a meal to assist the digestive process. Avoid exercise, sexual activity, study, or sleep should be avoided for an hour after a meal. But, if required, you can relax lying on your left side to encourage the proper function of the right nostril which will in turn encourage good digestion.

11.   Avoid wasting food which has been served to you. Serve yourself only the quantity that you require to avoid wasting food.

12.   After sunset do not eat foods that produce kapha, for example, yogurt and sesame.

13.   Do not eat anything within two hours of retiring for the night.

The modern scientists have also suggested the food combination. It is as follows:

1.   Eat acid fruits and starch at separate meals.

2.   Eat protein foods and carbohydrate foods at separate meals.

3.   Eat but one concentrated protein food at a meal.

4.   Eat protein foods and acid fruits at separate meals.

5.   Eat fat and protein food at separate meals.

6.   Eat sugar and protein food at separate meals.

7.   Eat starch and sugar at separate meals.

8.   Eat melons alone.

9.   Take milk alone.

10.   Acid fruits, fat, sugar and carbohydrate can be eaten together.

11.   Starch, fat and carbohydrate can be at a meal.

12.   Protein food and starch can be taken together.

I have included a chart on the constitution and the doshas so that it becomes easier for you to determine your personality type and typical dosha traits. This will also help you to follow the correct form of diet, which is best suited for you.

NO.		VATA	PITTA	KAPHA
1	Frame	thin	moderate	large
2	Weight	low	moderate	heavy
3	Skin	dry, rough, cool, brown and dark	soft, oily, warm and yellowish	thick, oily, cool, pale and fair
4	Hair	black and dry	soft, oily, yellow and early grey	thick, oily, dark or light
5	Teeth	protruding, spaces between	moderate, soft and bleeding gums	strong, white and well formed

		teeth, gums emaciated		
6	Eyes	small, dry, active, brown or black	sharp, grey or yellow	big, attractive, blue, thick eyelashes
7	Appetite	varied, low	good, sharp	slow, steady
8	Tendency to contract diseases	nervous disorders, pain of any kind	diseases of heat, infection	retention of water, diseases of kapha
9	Thirst	varied	excessive	slight
10	Bowel movement	dry, hard, constipated	soft, oily, loose	thick, oily, heavy, slow
11	Physical activity	very active	moderate	lethargic
12	Mind	restless, active, curious	aggressive, intelligent	calm, slow, receptive
13	Emotion	fearful, insecure, anxious	aggressive, irritable	greedy, attached, self-content
14	Faith	wavering, changeable	determined	steady, loyal
15	Memory	recent — good remote — poor	sharp	slow but prolonged
16	Dream	flying, jumping, running	fiery, angry, passionate swimming	watery, ocean,
17	Sleep	scanty, interrupted	little but sound	heavy, prolonged, excessive
18	Speech	fast, uninterrupted	sharp, clear, cutting	slow, monotonous, melodious

19	Tendency to spend	spends quickly	spends moderately, methodical	spends slowly, saves
20	Pulse rate	thready, feeble, moves like a snake	moderate, jumps like a frog	broad, slow, moves like a swan

For treating a patient the Ayurvedic physicians examine the above points and decide what medicine should be given.

IV   SPIRITUAL ENERGY MASSAGE

Before learning the techniques of Spiritual Energy Massage, you need to know more about spiritual energy. Though spiritual energy is a vast topic, here it is in a nut-shell.

KUNDALINI

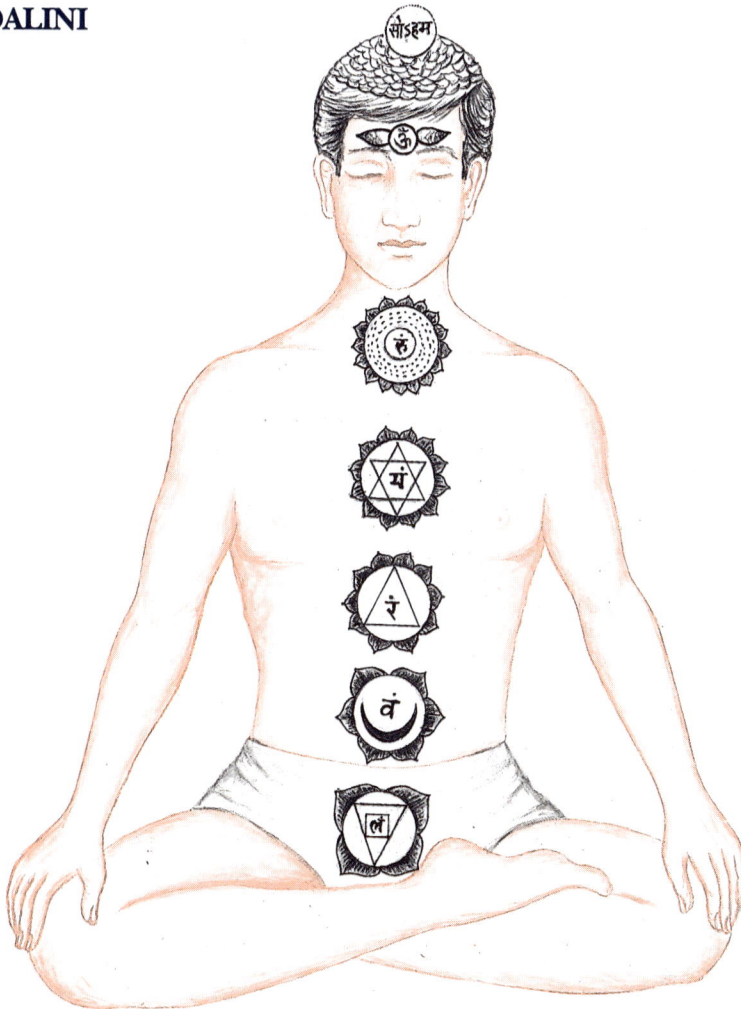

Fig. 27

The kundalini is a sleeping, dormant force which is like a coiled serpent at the base of the spinal column. This force (energy) is present in every human being. Kundal in Sanskrit means coil, therefore kundalini means the one that is coiled. The word kunda also means a cavity or a pit. Kundalini may also be derived from the root of the Sanskrit verb kund meaning burn and also from the noun kundalam meaning the one that is coiled. It is situated at the root of the spine, at the perineum (germinal gland) in the male which is between the urinary and the excretory organs. In the female it is located at the base of the uterus, in the cervix. It is symbolized by a shining serpent coiled three and a half times, with its tail in its mouth, lying as if asleep. The point where this energy lies is called the mooladhara chakra, the static support of the entire body and all its creative energy forces. This energy is the highest manifestation of consciousness in the human body and represents the creative force of the world as manifested in the human being. The kundalini is the embodiment of all powers and forms and is the seat of all physical and mental manifestations. It is the fountainhead of energy and knowledge and is not an object of visualization, but a subtle entity in the form of light (Figure 27).

The awakening of the kundalini involves rigorous training in terms of yogic asanas, pranayama, kriya yoga, and meditation. The actual forcing of the prana into the seat of the kundalini enables the energy to move upwards through various other centers situated in the central nervous canal to the brain. This awakening is akin to stimulating the silent areas of the brain.

The kundalini, like any force, has positive and negative aspects. It can also be interpreted as male and female. The awakening of this energy evolves a human being on a physical, mental and spiritual level. The raising of the kundalini brings forth a union between the two aspects mentioned earlier, which are also represented by Shiva and Shakti, male and female respectively. The awakening of the kundalini takes the human being onto a different level of consciousness and this improves the quality of experiences and perceptions of life. On the physical level too, one can expect changes. A change in voice may occur along with a change in body odor and hormones.

CHAKRAS

The kundalini is embodied where the concepts of time and space are nonexistent. This power is believed to arrive from the unconscious plane and move up through different phases until it unites with the supreme consciousness or what is otherwise called shiva. This energy passes through channels called chakras. The vital energy or the vital fire in the body is organized around specific centers which are not a part of the physical body but belong to the causal body. But they do correspond to the various plexuses in the human body. These specific centers are the chakras that help to organize the physical body although they cannot be perceived by means of the bodily senses and organs. The word chakra literally means 'circle or wheel' but in yogic terms it can be interpreted as a 'whirlpool' or 'vortex'. These chakras have particular rates of vibration. People experience chakras as circular movements because the chakras are vortices of psychic energy. The unconscious state lies in the mooladhara chakra. The supreme consciousness is in the sahasrara chakra which is in the crown of the head.

Active energy is distributed through the chakras as well as through an intricate network in the human body. This network is comprised of nadis which are channels that help the flow of consciousness. The word nadi actually means flow. About 72,000 nadis are believed to be distributed all over the body. Out of these, only three are vital for the flow of prana: ida, pingala, and sushumna. Each one controls different processes. Ida is in charge of the mental processes, pingala of the vital processes and the sushumna the awakening of the spiritual consciousness. They may thus be considered as mental, pranic and spiritual forces respectively. All the three nadis start at the mooladhara and end at the sahasrara, in the process of which they meet at each of the other chakras. The ida flows on the left and the pingala flows on the right of the spinal column while the sushumna flows up the central column, directly. The ida and the pingala do not operate simultaneously. On observing your nostrils you may notice that while you breathe through one, the other is blocked. Investigations show that if your left nostril is flowing, then the right side of your brain is activated and vice versa for the right nostril. This enables the nadis to control the various events of life and consciousness.

The chakras, located in the spinal column, distribute impulses. The uppermost chakra, however, is at the top of the head. In order to understand spiritual evolution and transformation, one should understand the chakras fully. The energy focused in the chakras is what determines personality and level of consciousness in the individual.

Sickness is always a physical expression of spiritual discord, which can also be dealt with on a subtler plane. Seven organs correspond to the seven chakras. The chakras are the connections between the energy body and the physical body and they are also connected to the kundalini force through the spine. The energetic quality of the chakras is purely a subtle vibration and is the source of our life energy.

Each of these chakras has a distinct color, sound and form. When the breath passes through them, each chakra focuses its own momentum and energy through nerve currents. Each of these currents influences the construction of the body corresponding to the particular center which is active at that time. For example, if breath is in the earth center, then the solidity of the body is influenced. Every chakra has a given number of nerve currents and these are symbolized by lotus petals. The chakras have graphic symbol colors as well as their element colors. For the massage it is essential to remember that the colors of the chakras used in meditation are the colors of the elements of the respective chakras and not the colors of the graphic symbols.

Mooladhara (Root) Chakra. The literal meaning of moola in Sanskrit is root or base. The Mooladhara in the male body is located in the perineum which is midway between the anus and the scrotum. It is connected with the testes and is responsible for carrying impulses through the nervous system. In the female, the chakra is located in the cervix. If the aspirant meditates on the mooladhara, he can have power over his speech, become a king among men and also a master of all learning. The other benefits are that he can be free of diseases and his personality will be cheerful. The symbol that represents mooladhara has four crimson lotus petals and a triangle facing downwards. The yellow square graphic shape represents the element earth or solid matter. The particular vibration with which this chakra rotates creates the sound lam, also known as a Bija Mantra. Breath stays in this chakra for a span of twenty minutes while flowing through the ida and pingala. Being the lowest of the chakras, it is associated with grosser emotions such as sensual enjoyment. While meditating on this chakra, a person is bound to experience a tremendous amount of sexual sensitivity. This is the main reason why the mooladhara chakra is not the first chakra in the sequence for spiritual energy massage (Figure 28).

Swadhisthana (Sacrum) Chakra. This chakra is also involved with the awakening of the kundalini. In Sanskrit swa means "one's very own"; adhisthana means "dwelling place"; swadhisthana means "one's own abode". Although the kundalini resides in the mooladhara chakra, in a sleeping state, its actual home is in the swadhisthana chakra. The exact location of this chakra is at the base of the spinal column at the level of the tailbone and the coccyx. You can feel it as a small bulb, bony in structure, a little above the anus. Anatomically, in both the male and the female, it is situated very close to the mooladhara. One who meditates on this chakra, it is believed, gets liberated from all internal enemies and lower forms of energy like lust, greed, anger, passion, sexual desires and fantasies, depression, procrastination, lethargy, and so on. The other psychic qualities that can be attained are a sudden awakening of intuitive knowledge, a loss of the fear of water and an awareness of astral entities around us (Figure 29).

Diseases related to the fluid systems in the body can be taken care of by focusing on this chakra. Herpes is one such ailment. A flash of yellow light during meditation indicates the energy of the mooladhara chakra whereas a blue light indicates the energy of the swadhisthana. Swadhisthana is represented by a six-petalled lotus which is orange-red or vermilion in color and its shape is of a half-moon. The element is water and the color is bluish. The graphic shape is semicircular and its force is contraction. It governs the sense of taste. Breath remains in this chakra for sixteen minutes while flowing through the ida and pingala. The bija mantra vam is the sound created by the vibration of this chakra.

Manipura (Solar Plexus) Chakra. In Sanskrit Manipura means "city of jewels". The word actually has two parts, mani which means jewel and pura which means city. This chakra is considered to be an important chakra in the process of the awakening of the kundalini, because it is the center of qualities like will, achievement, energy, and dynamism. The manipura chakra is located on the inner wall of the spinal column, just behind the navel. The manipura chakra is related anatomically to the solar plexus and controls the regulation of heat in the body. By meditating on this chakra, the aspirant will gain the power to create as well as destroy, lose the fear of fire, acquire hidden treasures, gain knowledge of one's body, and freedom from diseases. It also gives the aspirant the ability to withdraw energy to the sahasrara chakra. This chakra is symbolized by a yellow ten-petalled lotus. The form and graphic shape is a triangle pointing upward. Its element is fire, its color is red, and it governs the sense of sight. Manipura is responsible for the cleansing of the various systems of the body. Meditating on this chakra helps in the correct diagnosis of diseases and also helps the sweat glands, lungs, bowels, and kidneys to function well. The color of this chakra is red and the sound vibration is the bija mantra ram. The breath remains in this center for twelve minutes while flowing through the ida and pingala.(Figure 30).

Anahata (Heart) Chakra. The chakra is associated with the heart which is a throbbing, vibrating organ that beats with a constant rhythm. Anahata means unbeaten. This chakra is situated on the inner wall of the spinal column, just behind the center of the chest. Though it is associated with the heart, it should not be misinterpreted as the biological heart itself. The nature of this chakra is way beyond the physiological plane. Meditating on this chakra can help the aspirant to develop latent artistic talents and gain complete emotional balance. The awakening of this chakra brings about a constant feeling of optimism and also a sense of detachment to all worldly possessions. A person who has reached the anahata chakra stage develops a strong sense of touch which can heal the ailing. That person also becomes very sensitive to the feelings of the people around him. The anahata chakra has twelve shining crimson colored petals. Its color, however, is smoky and is symbolized by two intersecting triangles, each pointing in opposite directions. Its element is air and it governs the sense of touch. The graphic shape is a circle and its force is motion. The vibration of the sound is the bija mantra yam. While flowing through the ida and pingala, breath remains in the anahata for eight minutes. Emotional problems can be controlled and eliminated by meditating on this chakra (Figure 31).

Vishuddhi (Throat) Chakra. The harmonizing and purifying of all opposites in existence are at the center of vishuddhi chakra. Shuddhi in Sanskrit means to purify. This chakra is situated behind the pit of the throat and is in the cervical plexus. Meditation on this chakra helps the aspirant to develop a keen sense of hearing which is through the mind and not on the physiological plane, namely, the ears. This chakra is responsible for receiving thought vibrations from other people. The other powers include complete knowledge of the scriptures along with an awareness of the past, present, and future. This chakra is symbolized by a circle and sixteen purple lotus petals. The element of the vishuddhi is space, its color is blue, and it governs the sense of hearing. Its force is pervasion and breath remains in this chakra for four minutes while flowing through the ida and pingala. The vishuddhi is the refining center that controls the secret of youth and rejuvenation (Figure 32).

Ajna (Inner Eye) Chakra. The ajna chakra helps to bridge the gap between the guru (preceptor) and his disciples. The word ajna in Sanskrit means command (monitoring center). This chakra is located directly behind the eyebrow center in the brain. Since the exact location is difficult to find, the aspirant normally meditates on the eyebrow center. Development of the ajna chakra can bring about the attainment of knowledge without the help of the senses. With the awakening of this chakra, ficklemindedness of the individual disappears, making place for the purified higher intelligence and intuitive knowledge. The ajna is represented by a two-petalled lotus and has an intangible color. Its element is the mind. The vibration of this chakra is the bija mantra om. This chakra is believed to transcend all the gross elements, hence it is on the subtler plane (Figure 33).

Bindu Visarga Chakra. This chakra, which is the source of all creation, is actually beyond the realm of conventional experience. Therefore very little has been written about it. The literal meaning of the word bindu is "a point or a drop" but bindu visarga would accurately mean "falling of the drop". It is located at the back of the head at the shikha or choti, where some Hindu brahmins grow a longer tuft of hair. The bindu visarga is symbolized by the crescent moon and a white drop at the top indicating the flow of nectar to the vishuddhi chakra. This chakra is considered to be the seat of nectar which flows down to the vishuddhi chakra and spreads through the whole body. Some schools of yoga have not mentioned this chakra, but I have made a reference to it for your information.

Sahasrara (Crown). This is not a chakra as is often believed. It is really the point of culmination of the energy, rising through the different chakras. The word literally means a thousand. It is symbolized by a thousand-petalled lotus. The power of the chakras does not lie in them but resides in the sahasrara (Figure 34). It is actually the merging of prana and the supreme consciousness. This center transcends all logic and is totality itself. Union between the two forces, namely, shiva and shakti, takes place and indicates the starting point of a new experience. With this union the path of self-realization begins. It marks the death of individual awareness or the experience of name and form. The merging of the two forces creates nothingness and absolute silence. Different religions have their own terminology to describe this experience.

As mentioned earlier, the raising of the kundalini involves self-discipline, controlled diet, practice of yogasanas, and so on. This method is long and tedious. There is, however, an easy and succinct technique which involves blowing into this fire of primal energy with complete faith, purity of mind, thought, word, and deed. The action is not that of literally blowing, but breathing in and out, concentrating on the kundalini. The mantra used is Soham, meaning 'I am He' (Sah meaning He, Aham meaning I). The intake of breath sounds like so, aham is chanted during exhalation. Apart from this breathing technique, a special kind of foot massage also helps the aspirant. This not only helps in meditation, but also in moving into a state of yoga nidra. Yoga nidra should be done after you have completed the massage.

CHAKRAS AND THE ENDOCRINE GLANDS

The chakras are related to the endocrine glands. If the person concerned meditates with the knowledge of the situation of these glands, then the benefits attained are tremendous (Figure 35).

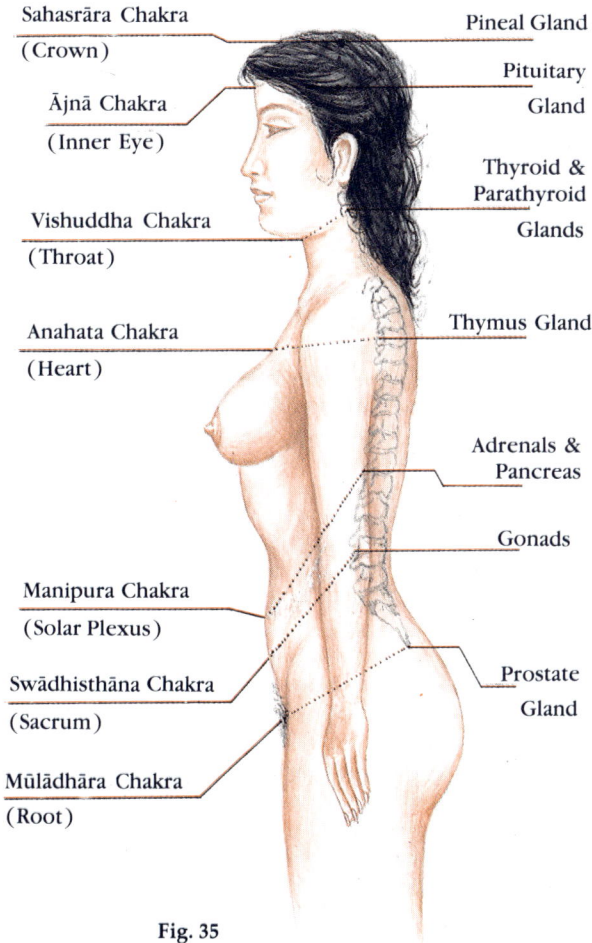

Sahasrāra Chakra
(Crown)

Pineal Gland

Pituitary
Gland

Ājnā Chakra
(Inner Eye)

Thyroid &
Parathyroid
Glands

Vishuddha Chakra
(Throat)

Anahata Chakra
(Heart)

Thymus Gland

Adrenals &
Pancreas

Gonads

Manipura Chakra
(Solar Plexus)

Swādhisthāna Chakra
(Sacrum)

Prostate
Gland

Mūlādhāra Chakra
(Root)

Fig. 35

CHAKRAS IN THE BODY

Endocrine glands are situated at various points in the human body and secrete chemical substances into the blood stream which have a great effect on the body and the mind. The endocrine glands consist of the pineal, pituitary, thyroid, thymus, adrenal and pancreas, gonads (ovaries in women and testes in men), and prostate glands.

Pineal Gland. This master gland of the body is situated at the center of the brain. It influences all the other glands that have been mentioned. It is associated with the sahasrara (crown) chakra, which is the center of supreme consciousness in an individual. Shashakasana (the hare posture) helps to stimulate the pineal gland which aids in concentration and calmness of the mind. The ideal time for meditation is from midnight to 3 a.m.

Pituitary Gland. This gland hangs by a short stalk in the front portion of the brain, just behind the trikuti. The pituitary gland controls all other glands. It enhances the quality of thinking. This gland corresponds to the ajna chakra.

Thyroid Gland. This gland, situated in the center of the neck, is related to the vishuddhi (throat) chakra. It controls the metabolic rate of the body. If the gland secretes thyroxin in excess, it results in the loss of weight, nervousness, extreme anxiety, quarrelsome nature, and sleeplessness. In order to balance the secretion one should practice sarvangasana (shoulder stand) and matsya mudra (fish posture). The combination of these two postures, repeated three times, squeezes and stretches the thyroid gland giving it a complete massage which enhances its health.

Thymus Gland. The thymus gland is near the heart and is, therefore, related to the anahata (heart) chakra. This gland controls the immune system of the body. Some diseases are a result of a weak thymus gland. Bhujangasana (cobra posture) strengthens the thymus gland and cures any weakness that exists in the upper part of the body.

Adrenal and Pancreas Glands. The manipura (solar plexus) chakra, associated with the adrenal glands, is located like two little caps on the top of the kidney. Adrenal glands control sudden bursts of energy, especially due to danger and stress. Tension is a result of excess adrenaline being secreted by the glands. This leads to high blood pressure, heart disease, ulcers, cancer, depression, and many other ailments. Shavasana helps to balance the adrenal glands and remove intensive stress. One can practice shavasana for about 10 minutes daily to balance the adrenal glands.

Gonads (ovaries in women and testes in men). Gonads are related to the swadhisthana chakra. Undersecretion of the testes and ovaries leads the person to become cruel and dogmatic. Gomukhasana (cow's face posture) pressurizes the chakra and cures its weakness.

Prostate Gland. It is related to the mooladhara chakra. It controls the flow of urine. Oversecretion of this gland causes a sense of hopelessness in life. The best cure for this is janushirsasana (head to knee—inverted).

The charts that follow show the chakras, their locations, color, sound, power, force, element, graphic shape, symbol etc., at a glance.

The first chart shows you the name of the chakra, the corresponding organ, plexus and the endocrine glands.

NO.	NAME OF CHAKRA	ORGAN	PLEXUS	ENDOCRINE GLAND
1	Mooladhara—Root	perineum	terrancon	prostate
2	Swadhisthana—Sacral	spleen	fluidal	gonads (ovaries and testes)
3	Manipura—Navel	navel	igneous	adrenals and pancreas
4	Anahata—Heart	chest	solar	thymus
5	Vishuddhi—Throat	throat	sidereal	thyroid
6	Ajna—Inner Eye	eyebrow center	lunar	pituitary
7	Sahasrara—Crown	head	multi-propensive	pineal

The second chart shows you the element, the power, force and the corresponding senses.

NO.	ELEMENT	POWER	FORCE	SENSES
1	earth	energy	solidity	smell
2	water	faith	counteraction	taste
3	fire	knowledge	expansion	sight
4	air	love	motion	touch
5	space	receiving	pervasion	hearing
6	mind	sending	thinking	—
7	—	wisdom	—	—

The third chart has the symbol, graphic shape, petals, duration of breath, sound and Yogasanas.

NO.	SYMBOL	GRAPHIC SHAPE	COLOR	PETALS	DURA-TION	SOUND	YOGA ASANAS
1	triangle apex down	square	yellow	4	20 min	LAM	Janushirs-asana
2	half moon	semi-circle	bluish	6	16 min	VAM	Gomukh-asana
3	triangle apex upward	triangle apex upward	red	10	12 min	RAM	Mayur-asana
4	inter-secting triangles apexes up & down	circle	smoky	12	8 min	YAM	Bhujang-asana
5	circle	space	blue	16	4 min	HAM	Sarvang-asana & Matsya Mudra
6	—	—	clear	32	—	OM	Sadhana
7	—	—	—	1000	—	SO HAM	Shashank-asana

TECHNIQUES OF SPIRITUAL ENERGY MASSAGE

The awakening of the kundalini is quite a long and tedious journey because it involves a lengthy procedure of yogasanas, pranayama, meditation, and so on. But I do a special kind of foot massage which also helps to raise the energy of the kundalini. This massage is helpful for those aspirants who use the mantra soham. I have had personal experience, because I practice it on myself everyday, before my meditation.

In my massage techniques, I use both reflexology and ayurvedic massage. This particular technique also helps the person to go into yoga nidra. I use pressure on certain points on the soles of my feet and also rotate my thumbs on them for the desired effect. I have observed that it benefits me tremendously in my meditation.

Spiritual energy massage techniques include the seven chakras (perineum, sacral, navel, chest, throat, forehead, and head) which help to regulate important processes connected with the body's metabolism. In case of any illness, insufficient interaction is taking place between these organs due to disharmony in the realm of energy on the

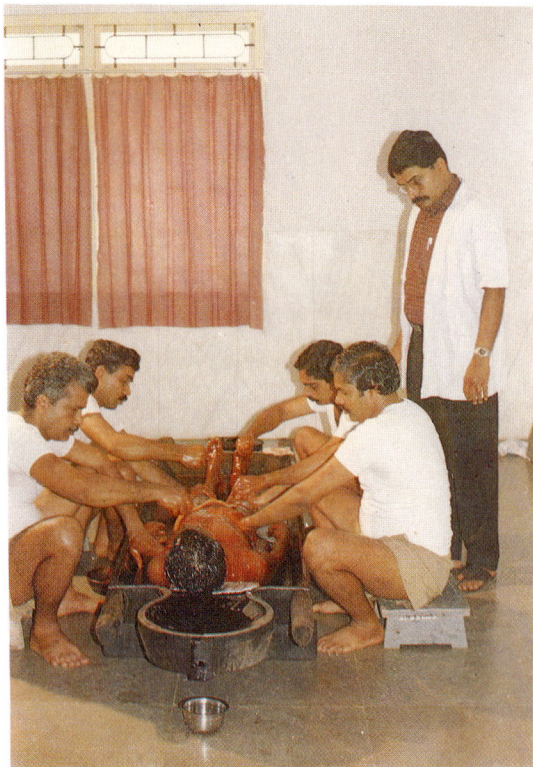

38.   Pizhichil (Squeezing)

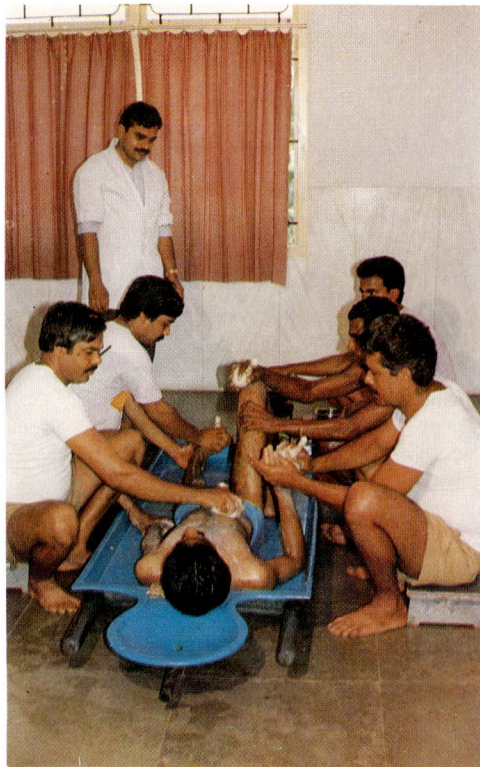

39.   Navarakkizhi (Bundle of specially cooked rice)

40.   Dhara (Flow)

41.   Shirovasti (Head cleansing)

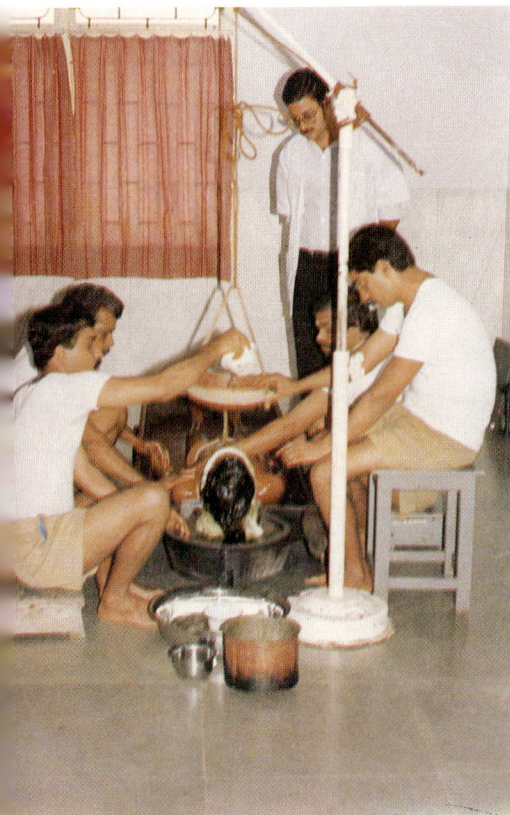

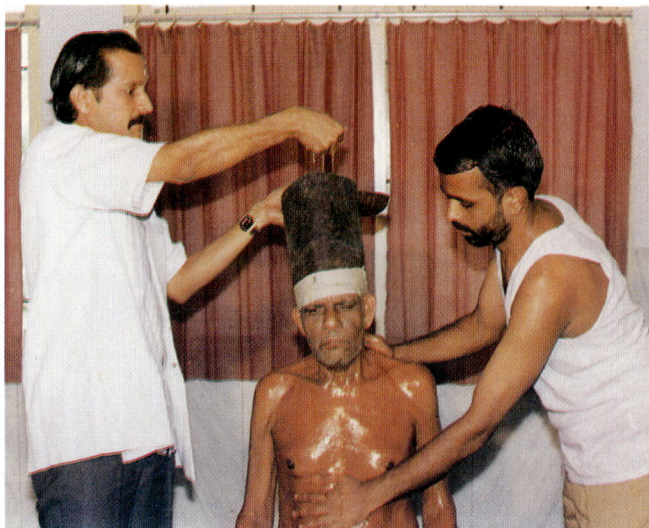

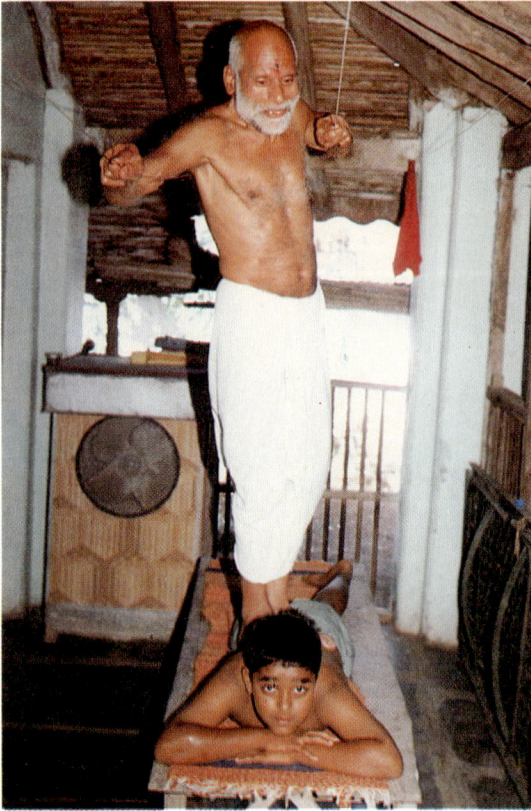

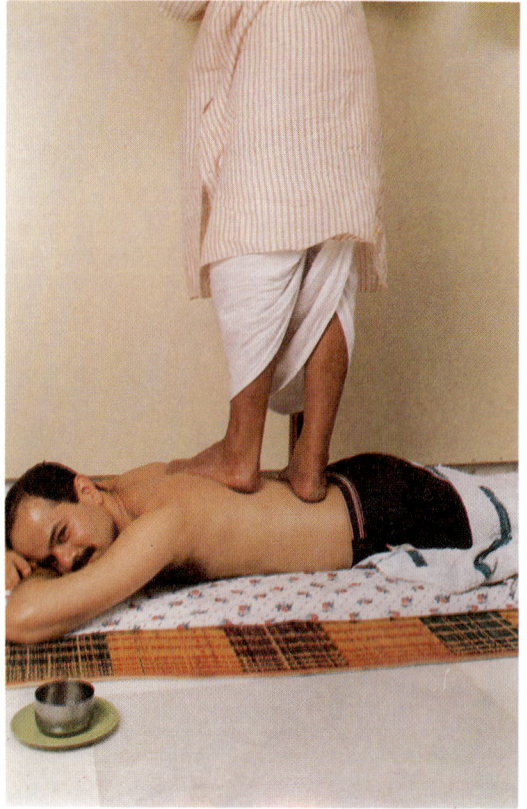

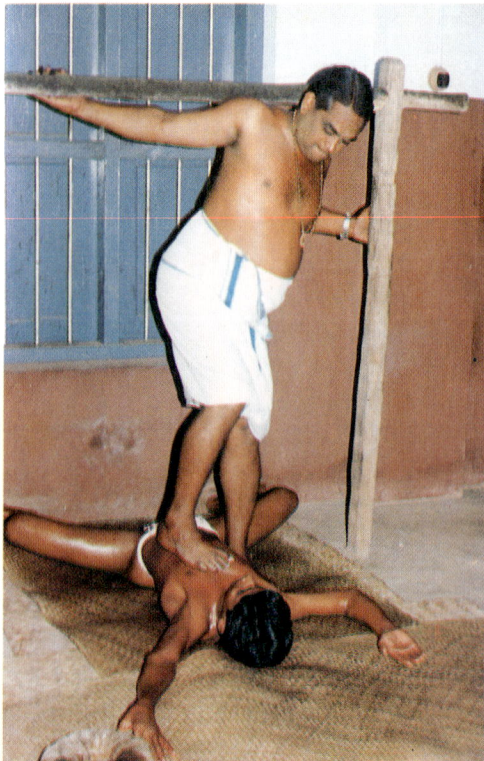

42. Massage with Legs

43. Massage with Legs

44. Massage with Legs

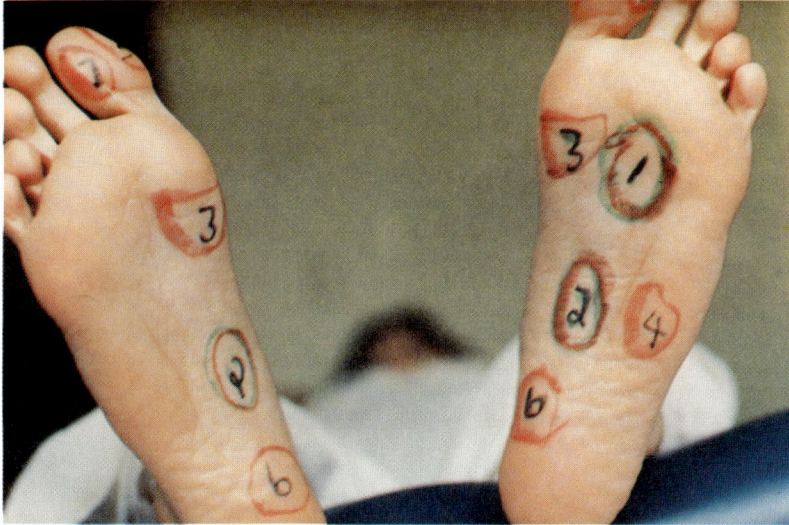

46. Spiritual Energy Massage Chakra points
     on both the soles

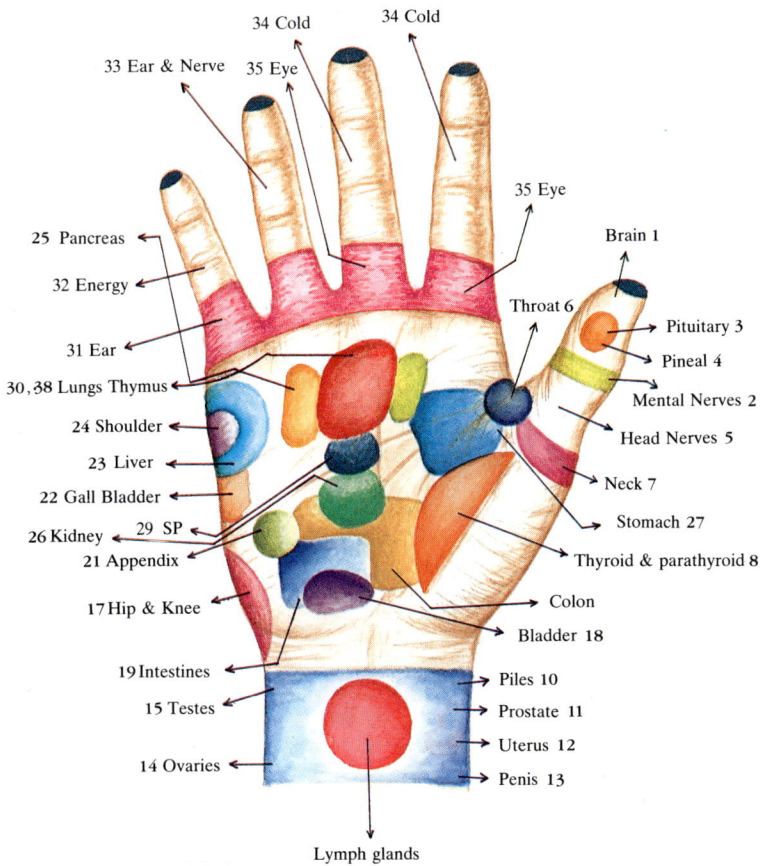

34 Cold

34 Cold

33 Ear & Nerve

35 Eye

35 Eye

Brain 1

25 Pancreas

Throat 6

Pituitary 3

32 Energy

Pineal 4

31 Ear

Mental Nerves 2

30, 38 Lungs Thymus

Head Nerves 5

24 Shoulder

Neck 7

23 Liver

22 Gall Bladder

Stomach 27

26 Kidney   29 SP

Thyroid & parathyroid 8

21 Appendix

17 Hip & Knee

Colon

Bladder 18

19 Intestines

Piles 10

15 Testes

Prostate 11

Uterus 12

14 Ovaries

Penis 13

Lymph glands

Fig. 39

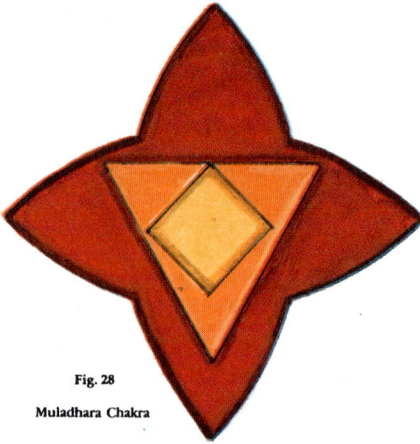

Fig. 28

Muladhara Chakra

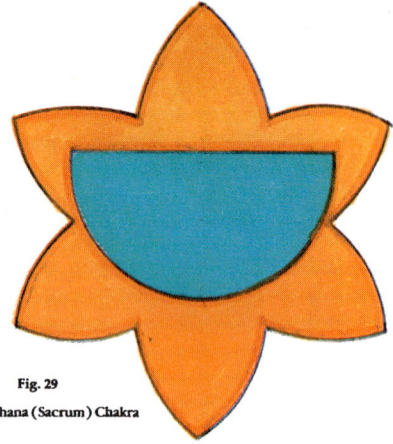

Fig. 29

Swadhisthana (Sacrum) Chakra

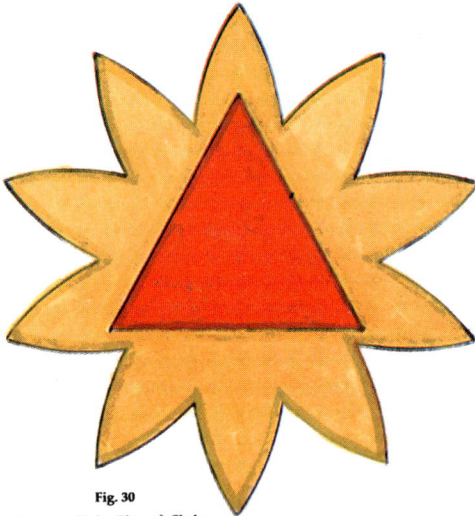

Fig. 30

Manipura (Solar Plexus) Chakra

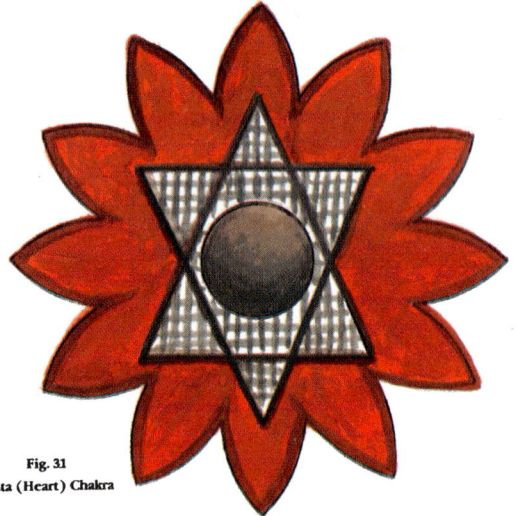

Fig. 31

Anahata (Heart) Chakra

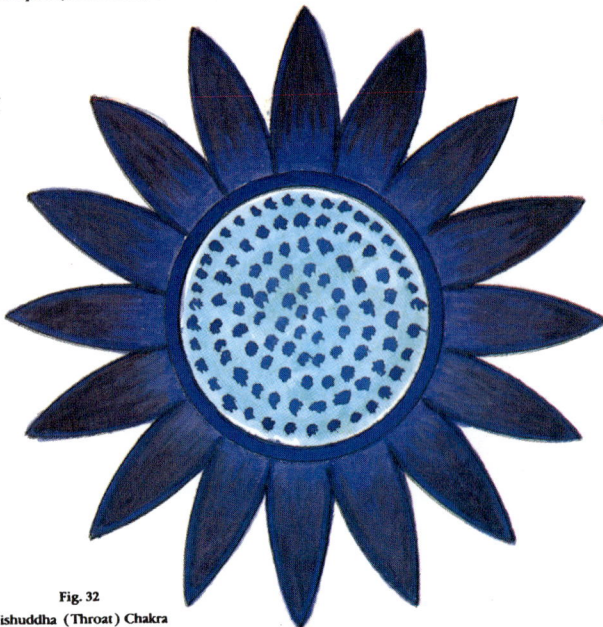

Fig. 33

Ajna (Inner Eye) Chakra

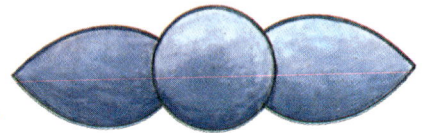

Fig. 32

Vishuddha (Throat) Chakra

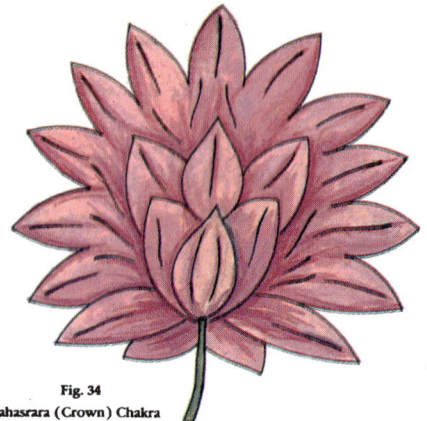

Fig. 34

Sahasrara (Crown) Chakra

subtler plane. This can be identified due to the obstruction in the energy of one or more chakras. These minor or even major ailments can be handled with this simple method of treatment.

With the help of the aura, the invisible bioplasmic body that surrounds the physical body, one can scan the clinical status from its radiation. Along with other illnesses, blockades, congestions, drainage, and forms of obsessions and possessions can be identified. In yoga each color has its specific vibration that corresponds to each chakra on the subtler plane. These colors are projected in the aura of the patient and any disturbances caused in any of the chakras will have a detrimental effect on the sensitive vibrations of the aura and its entirety.

I have personally experienced the conversion of knowledge to wisdom by means of this massage for spiritual energy. I perceived from the subconscious, with a great sense of peace, that this could be a holistic method of healing. The sahasrara (crown) chakra contains all the colors of the spectrum, but in the final stage of spiritual evolution all chakras emanate the purest white light which is as clear as a diamond. This is the expression of the attainment of perfection. In spiritual energy massage, we make use of these colors and different reflexology points in order to unfold and stimulate the existing healing processes in the human body.

The vibrations that exist in life are in the forms of colors, sounds, fragrances, and symbols, and all this is a mere rotation of energy. Energy can never be lost. It only gets converted into another form of vibration. Einstein's theory of relativity says that all matter is vibration and the wholeness of creation becomes comprehensible and becomes inverted. Above is below, positive is negative, inhaling is exhaling and death is life. Energy is never lost, it merely transforms into another form of vibration. The vibration of each chakra can be harmonized and intensified through the energy radiation of the corresponding colors, sounds, fragrances, symbols, elements, graphic shapes, and so on. The synchronization of these factors helps the patient to maintain sound health physically, mentally and spiritually. For example, green color does not correspond to any particular chakra, but it has very important therapeutic qualities. It relaxes and harmonizes the body on the whole.

One important factor to observe is that spiritual energy massage should not start from the mooladhara chakra for a simple reason. The awakening of this chakra focuses on the increase in sexual desires and fantasies. For beginners, who may not know how to remedy the situation, may find it difficult to proceed from the mooladhara (root) chakra. Therefore we start from the anahata (heart) chakra. By massaging this chakra, the aspirant opens a sphere of emotion and an all-encompassing love envelops his/her entire being and helps to create an equilibrium. This helps in the development of the other chakras. The anahata chakra activates the manipura (solar plexus) chakra, then the vishuddhi (throat) chakra, the swadhisthana (sacrum) chakra, followed by the ajna (inner eye) chakra, the mooladhara (root) chakra and finally the sahasrara (crown) chakra. Thus the Yin Yang principle remains completely unimpaired and a balance between the physical and spiritual worlds is maintained. With this the aspirant can transform elementary driving force into genuine life energy.

Before starting the massage session make sure that the following requirements are fulfilled. Prepare and play an audio cassette with soothing music and the bija mantras corresponding to the chakras in their order of massage. The duration of each mantra should be in the following order: the mantra Yam for two and a half minutes, Ram for five minutes, Ham for five minutes, Vam for two and a half minutes, Om for five minutes, Lam for five minutes, and Soham for five minutes. As the mantras change, change the massage points accordingly. Make the symbols of each of the chakras on pieces of cloth with the corresponding colors of the chakras. Be sure to have incense sticks lighted throughout the session. Make spots of different colors: yellow, light blue, red, smoky grey,

CHAKRA REFLEXOLOGY POINTS

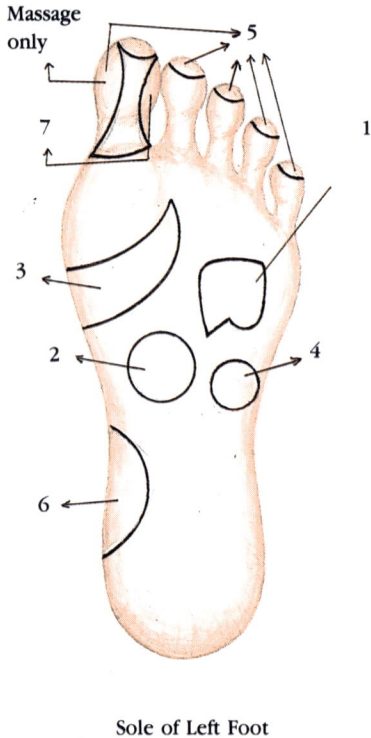

Massage only

Fig. 36

1. Heart (Anahata or Heart Chakra) Love

2. Solar Plexus (Manipura or Solar Plexus Chakra) Knowledge

3. Thyroid Gland (Vishuddha or Throat Chakra) Receiving

4. Adrenal Gland Spleen (Swādhisthāna or Sacrum Chakra) Faith

5. Pineal (Ājnā or Inner Eye Chakra) Sending

6. Prostate Gland Sacrum (Mūlādhāra or Root Chakra) Energy

7. Pituitary Gland (Sahasrara or Crown Chakra) Wisdom

Note: 1. Points 1 and 4 – only on Left Sole
       2. Massage point 5 only on outer side of the big toe of both feet.

Sole of Left Foot

and blue. Have ready cow's ghee (butter) in yellow, red, smoky grey, and blue colored bottles as well as in a transparent bottle. Have ready basil leaves and rose water. Make sure the ambience of the room is conducive for the massage session. The surroundings should be calm and quiet. Make use of the above-mentioned requirements because they are inter-connected and will help to bring the vibration of the chakras to their original harmony. The time required for the spiritual energy massage is about 30 minutes (Figure 36).

Anahata (Heart) Chakra (Photo 46). Have the patient/client lie down in a comfortable posture. Light the incense sticks so that the room becomes fragrant. Put a few drops of rose water in the patient's eyes and nose. Ask the patient to visualize smoky grey color. You may place on the patient's chest a similar colored piece of cloth with a symbol of two intersecting triangles with their apexes in opposite directions and a circle in the middle with twelve petals. By doing this, the expression of life synchronizes with the biological rhythm of the body. If the patient cannot visualize the smoky grey color, then ask the patient to concentrate on the similar colored spot. Play the cassette with the bija mantras in the background. The corresponding mantra for this chakra is Yam. Apply cow's ghee (butter) on the heart chakra point, which is directly below the last two toes on the left foot only. Massage this point with a circular movement for about two minutes; then press the point for about half a minute. The patient may experience a warm feeling and a pleasant pulsation during the treatment. When the mantra changes move to the next prescribed chakra.

Manipura (Solar Plexus) Chakra. Play the bija mantra Ram and place the symbol of a downward pointing triangle with ten petals on a red colored cloth on the navel of the patient. Ask the patient to visualize the color red. Keep the incense sticks lighted. Using cow's ghee (butter) from a red bottle, massage the solar plexus point which is in the pit of the arch of both the feet. Use circular movements on these points and massage each foot for two and a half minutes with pressure for a total of five minutes. The manipura is the focal point of primal knowledge and it also reflects all fears. The harmonious interaction of all the stimulation factors for this chakra eventually helps to dissolve all fears. In case the patient experiences pain during the massage of this chakra, do not stop, but continue, using steady pressure for the prescribed time. Having harmonized the vibrations, move on to the next chakra which is the vishuddhi (throat) chakra.

Vishuddhi (Throat) Chakra. Continue with playing the bija mantra Ham. Ask the patient to visualize blue color or concentrate with his eyes on the blue spot. Place on the patient the cloth symbol of a circle with holes and sixteen petals. Massage the vishuddhi chakra points on both the feet for two and a half minutes on each foot. The points are located on the inner rim of the ball of the feet. Use semicircular movements for this chakra. Diseases caused due to the throat chakra energy not being in harmony are difficulty in swallowing, chronic hoarseness, problems of the thyroid gland, and tonsillitis. Massage of this point helps the patient to purify the mind of unclean thoughts. The chakra harmonizes with the purification of the mental space.

Swadhisthana (Sacral) Chakra. Continue playing the bija mantra Vam on the cassette and keep the incense sticks lighted. For this chakra ask the patient to visualize a bluish color and place the symbol below the navel of the patient. The symbol consists of a semicircular bluish cloth with six petals. The point is situated straight below the little toe on the left foot only. Massage this point with cow's ghee from a blue bottle. Use the same circular movements for two minutes with steady pressure for half a minute. The patient may experience an intense sensation of warmth in the upper abdomen. Diabetes can be controlled by the massage of this chakra. The individual's blood sugar can be kept in check. This massage helps to increase an immense source of strength and faith.

Ajna (Inner Eye) Chakra. Continue playing the cassette in the background with the bija mantra Om. Have the patient lie still in the calm atmosphere without really concentrating on any particular color because the ajna has no tangible color or symbol. You can keep a basil leaf on the forehead between the eyebrows. Now using cow's ghee, massage the points of all the toes on both feet or only the outer rim of the big toes. Massage the points for a duration of two and a half minutes for each foot. These points are in the area of the sinus. If the harmony of this chakra is disturbed, it not only leads to a particular disease but may also affect a whole organ.

Mooladhara (Root) Chakra. For this chakra cover the anus and the genitals with a yellow, four-petalled piece of cloth with a triangle in the center with its apex below and a square in the center also with four petals. Play the bija mantra Lam in the background. Using cow's ghee from a yellow bottle, massage the points on the inner rim of the heel on both the feet for two and a half minutes for each foot. The seat of the most elementary vital force is this chakra. Unrealized or misguided sexual energy will manifest itself as a migraine headache or as a remarkably frequent bladder problem. With massage the patient can transform and become receptive and devoted toward the other partner. The vibrations created can make it possible for the root chakra to open so the energy can spiral its way up to the crown chakra.

Sahasrara (Crown) Chakra. Play the mantra So] [ham for this chakra. Ask the patient to visualize a bright light. Keep a tulsi or basil leaf on the brahma randhra. The massage of this chakra point opens up the highest center for energy. Again using cow's ghee (butter), massage the point which is on the inner side of the big toe. Using rotating movements, massage both points on both the feet for two and a half minutes each. Disharmony in this area of the uppermost chakra can affect all the elemental life processes. This chakra is the point of union between the body and soul. Cosmic information is received through the pituitary gland from where the impulses are passed onto the thymus gland that is connected to the heart chakra. These impulses are experienced as emotions. If the thymus gland is in a state of perfect harmony with the heart chakra we can transform everything into a sense of universal love.

Though this massage can be done by one's self, the pleasure will be greater if the massage is done by another person. Through daily experience, the recipient may experience yoga nidra.

APPENDIX A

Acupressure and Reflexology

Nature has provided our bodies with an in-built mechanism to maintain our health and take care of ailments and diseases that might plague us. Various points situated all over the body correspond to various organs in the human body. The manipulation, stimulation, or massage of these points help to tackle a particular ailment as already mentioned regarding shiatsu. Next is discussion of two more therapies, one from the East and one from the West.

ACUPRESSURE

Whenever we experience pain or strain in a particular part of our body, our immediate reaction is to rub that area to get some relief. Acupressure has been derived from man's natural desire to rub, caress, or press any particular affected part to obtain relief. These points are located all over the body and correspond to various organs. If pressure is exerted on any point on that meridian corresponding to that organ, the pain can be handled.

In ancient India, elephant trainers are said to have used sharp objects to train the animals. They used these instruments without much observation as to why the animal would settle down so quickly. Gradually they realized that it was due to the pressure exerted on certain points behind the ear. This made some intelligent people think about the same cause and effect relationship with respect to humans. Gradually, physicians of Ayurveda adopted this method of treating their patients. Sushruta is said to have been the very first one to have made use of this technique in surgery, wherein he could sedate a patient before surgery and revive him after surgery by manipulating certain points on the body. It is believed, according to one theory, that acupressure and acupuncture originated in India, and later spread to Egypt, Central Asia, China, and other Eastern countries through Buddhist monks. The Chinese, however, believe it to be their own science and claim that it is more than 5000 years old. Whatever the theories and opinions may say, the Chinese have definitely made acupressure and acupuncture well known in the whole world.

The word acu means to remove or take out the toxins and other unwanted waste materials from the body. Therefore acupressure means taking out disease-infested matter from the body with the help of pressure. The idea that prevention is better than cure should be given much more importance, like the Chinese do. Today in India, people use

ACUPRESSURE POINTS

Fig. 40

RIGHT SOLE

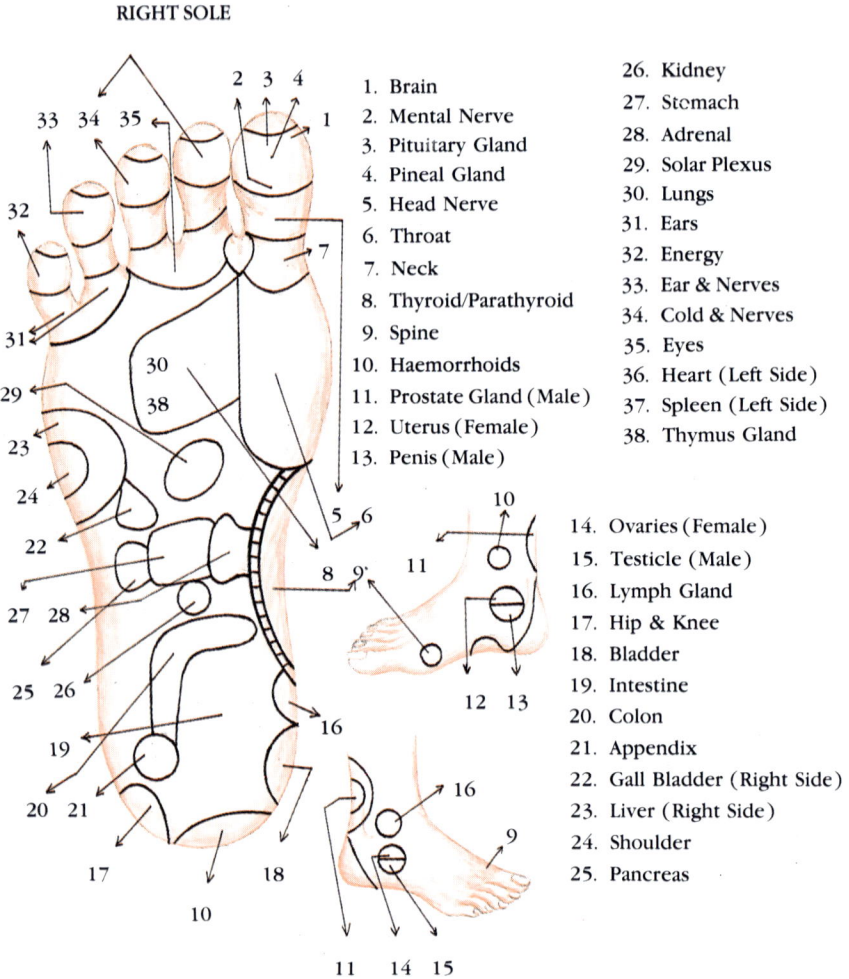

1. Brain
2. Mental Nerve
3. Pituitary Gland
4. Pineal Gland
5. Head Nerve
6. Throat
7. Neck
8. Thyroid/Parathyroid
9. Spine
10. Haemorrhoids
11. Prostate Gland (Male)
12. Uterus (Female)
13. Penis (Male)

14. Ovaries (Female)
15. Testicle (Male)
16. Lymph Gland
17. Hip & Knee
18. Bladder
19. Intestine
20. Colon
21. Appendix
22. Gall Bladder (Right Side)
23. Liver (Right Side)
24. Shoulder
25. Pancreas

26. Kidney
27. Stomach
28. Adrenal
29. Solar Plexus
30. Lungs
31. Ears
32. Energy
33. Ear & Nerves
34. Cold & Nerves
35. Eyes
36. Heart (Left Side)
37. Spleen (Left Side)
38. Thymus Gland

acupressure to cure diseases. Historically, the foundation for making most therapies preventive rather than curative has already been laid, though it is being picked up very slowly today.

The meridians, fourteen of them, are similar to the shiatsu meridians and so are the points along these meridians. See the discussion of shiatsu for details. The masseur/masseuse who knows these meridians and points along them will have an advantage when doing massage because the patient can be relieved of aches and pains.

Each one of the fourteen meridians branches out into many subsidiary meridians. The area of influence of the main meridians increases due to the various subsidiary meridians. The meridian is actually the main force controlling that particular part of the body through which it passes. The disease may be anything but the treatment remains the same. Acupressure is, therefore, very simple and easy to practice.

In case of any ailment, only certain points on the meridian become inflamed corresponding to the affected organ. This is because these points act as controllers or regulators and check the flow of energy through the meridians. The movement or circulation of bioenergy flowing through the meridians can be rectified by the manipulation of certain points. The meridian and points are no longer painful when the disease is eliminated, therefore the affected organ and the meridian are interrelated.

Sometimes, in the case of certain diseases, no signs appear externally. A person may have a general feeling of weakness. Basic tests sometimes do not reveal the problem. In acupressure, it is possible to diagnose an ailment in its initial stage. This is done through the points which are painful when the patient is suffering from any ailment (Figures 39 & 40).

Acupressure considers the human body as a whole and strives to maintain the balance in the energies which flow through the body. According to theory, acupressure claims to relieve and cure most ailments with some exceptions. For example, acupressure can do nothing in cases of large gall stones, cancer, mature cataract, and kidney-stones. The success of this treatment depends upon factors like the duration of the disease, condition of the patient, and the extent of damage already caused. Acupressure, however, can be used along with other forms of treatment. It enhances the efficacy of the different systems and organs in the body. It helps to prevent a relapse of any disease. In short, acupressure can be used more as a preventive therapy than as a curative one. Another important benefit of this therapy is that it emphasizes the concept of touch, thus helping to build a relationship between the patient and the therapist.

The body is said to have an in-built mechanism to revitalize itself and relieve any kind of tension or discomfort that one may feel. I have explained how you can use these points to cure certain common ailments. For acupressure, the masseur/masseuse may use his/her hands or make use of instruments or gadgets made of either wood or metal.

These gadgets are grooved to facilitate the manipulation of the points and also to give the right amount of pressure.

General Treatment

Revitalization. The patient can feel refreshed by pressing the whole area, on both the palms, everyday for 13 minutes. Pressure should reach every square inch on the palm from the wrist to the tips of the fingers. A person can feel more energetic and younger by pressing in the middle of the forearm of the patient's right hand.

Control hunger. Press deeply on the three points on the ear for about 5 minutes half an hour before the meal. Keep the thumb behind the ear while applying pressure and breathe through the right nostril for 15 minutes.

Burns. Massage strongly in the middle of the front of the wrist. The burning sensation will be reduced considerably.

Keeping hair from turning grey or white. One can avoid the greying of hair and falling hair by rubbing the nails of eight fingers against each other for 10 minutes daily, 5 minutes in the morning and 5 minutes in the evening.

Corns. Massage the affected part with ice at night before retiring. Rub turpentine on it for two minutes and bandage it. In the morning the corn will come out without a problem. Continue rubbing turpentine daily for a period of three days.

Toothache. Find the fingertip that corresponds to the affected tooth. Press the tip of the finger continuously for 3 minutes. If the pain persists, continue the treatment for more time (Figure 37).

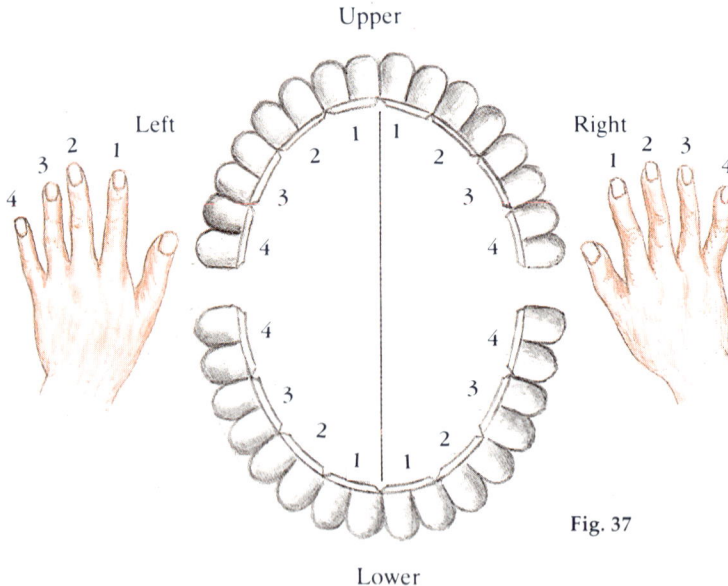

Fig. 37

TOOTHACHE

Backache. Rub hard between the thumb and the index finger to the middle of the wrist for 5 minutes. This will relieve the pain.

Pain in the legs. Roll the soles of the feet on a grooved wooden roller for a period of 3 minutes.

Chest pain. Press in the middle of the back of the forearm for 3 minutes.

Asthma. Rub from the middle of the chest to the sides for 5 minutes. Then press the joint in the middle of the dip on the neck for 1 minute.

Abdominal Ailments

Digestive system. To activate the digestive system, roll the soles of the feet on a grooved wooden roller for 5 minutes daily. This treatment is very useful for people over 45 years of age.

Constipation. Constipation can be avoided by pressing or rubbing the middle of the chin for 5 minutes daily before your morning routine.

Painless childbirth. Roll a grooved wooden roller vigorously on the back of both the arms of the expectant mother for 15 minutes daily for 15 days before her due date. Rub the back of both the palms from nail to wrist and the soles from nails to ankle continuously with metal combs for 10 minutes daily. If the mother goes into labor, let her hold the metal combs between the tips of her fingers including the thumb and the upper part of the palms. Press and release at intervals of 2 minutes on the back of the palm as shown in Figure 38. This exercise may be continued for 5 minutes. The woman will deliver within 30 minutes without any difficulty or feeling of tiredness. If she feels a slight pain during delivery, press on the inner side of the leg above the ankle for 2 minutes with a pause of 2 minutes. Continue this process until the baby is born. After the delivery if the woman has any discomfort and pain due to the accumulation of breast

TIPS OF LEGS AND PALMS

Fig. 38

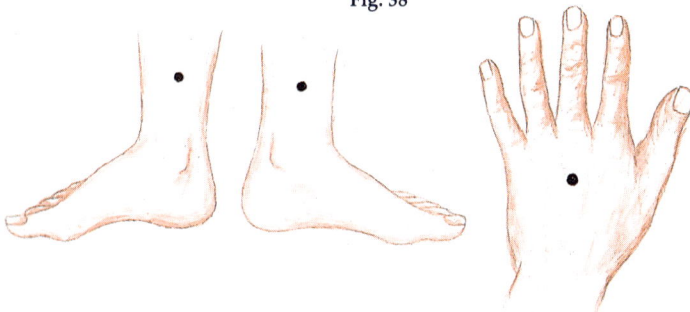

milk, press in the middle of the back of both the palms. The patient will be relieved immediately.

Obesity. Some people tend to put on excess weight after delivery due to a hormonal imbalance. If pressure on points 3, 4, 8, 11, 12, 13, 14, 15, 16, 25, 28, and 38 is given daily for 5 minutes from the day after the delivery, the patient will be able to maintain good health, both physically and mentally.

Nervous Disorders

Nervous tension. Clap your palms tightly and interlock your fingers. Press on the back of your hands with the fingers of the opposite hand. Do not separate the interlock. Repeat this for 3 minutes 4 times a day. Doing this exercise for 10 minutes before retiring for the night will ensure sound, undisturbed sleep.

Hysteria. Press on the inner side of the first joint of the thumb for 5 minutes. This will help the patient to calm down.

Fainting. Press on the inner side of the nail of the little finger. The patient will regain consciousness.

Sun-stroke, fainting and bleeding through the nose. Press the tips of all fingers and toes for 10 minutes and also press hard below the nose above the upper lip for 2 minutes. Induce the patient to breathe only through the left nostril, by blocking the right nostril.

REFLEXOLOGY (ZONE THERAPY)

Reflexology (zone therapy) originated in the United States some centuries ago. Dr. Fitzgerald developed it, but some writers claim that reflexology, like acupressure, has its roots in China. It is also said to have been discovered about 5000 years ago. What is reflexology (zone therapy) all about and how does it differ from acupressure?

This therapy is based on the theory and principle that the feet and hands are reflectors of the internal organs of the body. Therefore points in the area of the feet correspond to the different internal organs of the body. By way of stimulation, of any point on the foot, energy is transmitted through the nerves and this makes a direct change in the corresponding part of the body.

What really happens is that when about 72,000 nerve endings are stimulated, the energy flows through all the pathways which are not blocked or obstructed by deposits of toxins. In reflexology these toxins are called crystals. This flow of energy helps to directly attack and cause disintegration of this waste material (crystals) so that energy can flow freely again throughout the body. The free-flowing energy not only releases the crystals but also helps to eliminate tension and stress. The instant that happens, the circulation of blood to these areas increases, thus speeding up the body's own healing process.

In the course of precise palpation in the areas of these deposits, there may be pain and light to dark red discoloration. In extreme cases, blisters may also appear. When the body's immune system does not completely cure the ailments, they leave behind traces in the corresponding reflex zones. Reflexology zones contain terminal points or nerve endings that are directly connected to a distant organ or part of the body. Reflexive action of the nervous system, that transmits the impulses of all stimuli, takes place within the entire body. Insufficient functioning of the organs (kidneys, intestines, lungs, and skin) involved in the elimination of body wastes may also cause the depositing of the remaining metabolic waste products. When medicines are taken, we find pharmaceutical residue in the blood and in the cells of the body which form deposits of organic wastes at the nerve terminal points, particularly in close proximity of the spinal column.

Pain is not a disease. Pain is the clearest possible sign of a disturbance somewhere in the body. The body has no other means, other than pain, to direct attention to it. So in reality, pain is a blessing in disguise. Pain is our body's cry for help. Nowadays people do not walk or run along bumpy roads and on naturally uneven ground. When people would do that in the days gone by, it would act as an automatic masseur and the various points on the feet would be pressed. This would greatly reduce the possibility of disease and pain. But today, our lifestyles are such that we have to undergo a lot of pain before we can put our finger on the problem.

First and foremost palpate the nerve points to find out the areas of disturbance in the body. Ask the patient to lie down on his/her back, comfortably, with the feet slightly raised. Find the solar plexus (situated about a palm's breath above the navel in the hollow of the rib cage) which should not be cramped such that it hinders free breathing and thus impairs the functioning of the autonomous nervous system.

Give precise palpation for about an hour by applying oil to the patient's feet to enhance movement of the hands during the stimulation. Rotate the thumbs in a circular motion. Begin with large circles and slowly contract them towards the center of the area. Since the reflex zone of the solar plexus is the key to the autonomous nervous system, subconscious treatment starts from there. Stabilizing the solar plexus point results in an immediate loosening of the entire area. During palpation if there is any hardening of crystals or cramping, the patient may react with violent fits of crying. In such a case continue pressing and within a few minutes the patient will get relief. This treatment helps to loosen cramps and blockades. If there is serious hardening or reddish discoloration, extend the massage from two to five minutes.

The reflex zone pathways cross at the solar plexus. If the indication is in the left foot, the disturbance will be located on the right side of the body and vice versa. The reflex zones for the heart and spleen are in the left foot, whereas for the liver and gall bladder in the right foot. The spinal column, stomach, uterus, prostate gland, pituitary gland, and thyroid gland are aligned with the vertical body axis. They are radiated into both sides of the body and have reflex zones in both feet.

SKELETAL MASSAGE

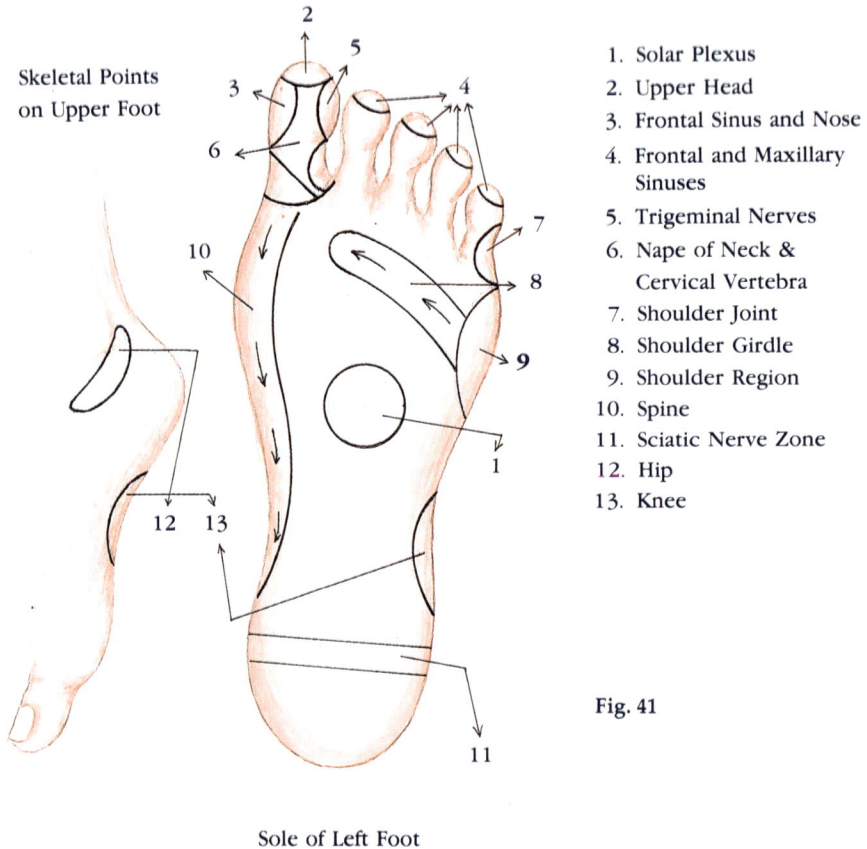

Skeletal Points
on Upper Foot

1. Solar Plexus
2. Upper Head
3. Frontal Sinus and Nose
4. Frontal and Maxillary
   Sinuses
5. Trigeminal Nerves
6. Nape of Neck &
   Cervical Vertebra
7. Shoulder Joint
8. Shoulder Girdle
9. Shoulder Region
10. Spine
11. Sciatic Nerve Zone
12. Hip
13. Knee

Fig. 41

Sole of Left Foot

The masseur/masseuse and the patient should have a mutual trust, which is the foundation of every healing process. First start with the left foot and examine the area of the upper head and then immediately take the other foot and do the same. Work is done from the toes to the heels in order to prevent an energy congestion from occurring in the body.

The three massage programs skeletal, digestive, and lymphatic. Between two massages, there should be a gap of 24 hours so that the body has enough time to eliminate waste matter that has been loosened. The deciding factor of massage is not so much the force but the transmission of warmth and life energy. Due to this, true communication from body to body and soul to soul needs to be established.

Massage Instructions

1.   Let the patient lie comfortably on the back with feet slightly raised.

2.   The masseur should keep a towel and oil ready.

3.   Every massage begins with the solar plexus points, simultaneously on the left and right foot, along the soles, along the sides, and on the top of the feet all the way to the heels. Without exception, all massages are brought to a close with a relaxation program, by exerting gentle pressure on the lymphatic area. The arrows in the illustrations indicate the direction of massage so that the pressure of the rotating thumb always tends to move upwards towards the center.

Guidelines for Massage

1.   Skeletal program. This involves massage in the following order: solar plexus, upper head, frontal sinus and nose, maxillary, trigeminal nerves, nape of the neck and

DIGESTIVE MASSAGE

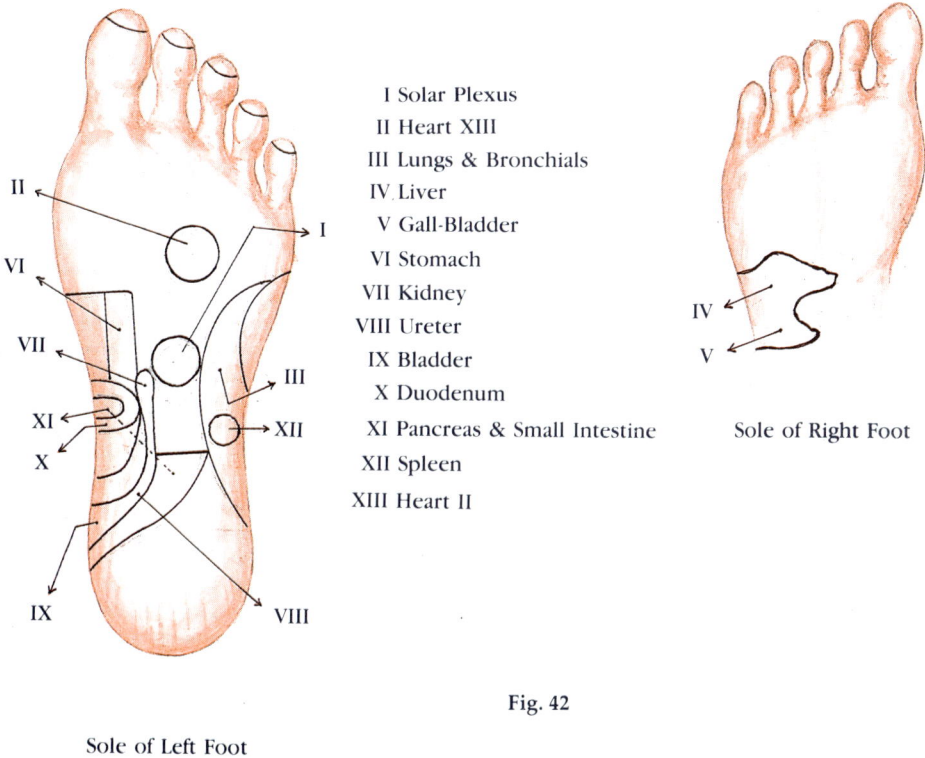

I Solar Plexus

II Heart XIII

III Lungs & Bronchials

IV Liver

V Gall-Bladder

VI Stomach

VII Kidney

VIII Ureter

IX Bladder

X Duodenum

XI Pancreas & Small Intestine

XII Spleen

XIII Heart II

Sole of Right Foot

Fig. 42

Sole of Left Foot

cervical vertebra, shoulder joint, shoulder girdle, shoulder region, spinal column, sciatic nerve, hip, knee, and relaxation, as shown in Figure 41.

2. Digestive program. This program includes the solar plexus, heart (to all patients, except those who have low blood pressure), lungs and bronchial tubes, liver, gall bladder, stomach, kidney, ureter, bladder, intestine, and duodenum, pancreas and small intestine, spleen, heart (in case of high blood pressure, massage prior to relaxation) and relaxation. Figure 42 gives key points for digestive massage.

3. Lymphatic program. This involves the solar plexus, pituitary gland, parathyroid gland, ears, eyes, thyroid gland, uterus/prostate gland, ovaries/grounds, tonsils, equilibrium, chest region, inguen channel, lymphatic zones, hemorrhoids, and relaxation. These points are shown in Figure 43.

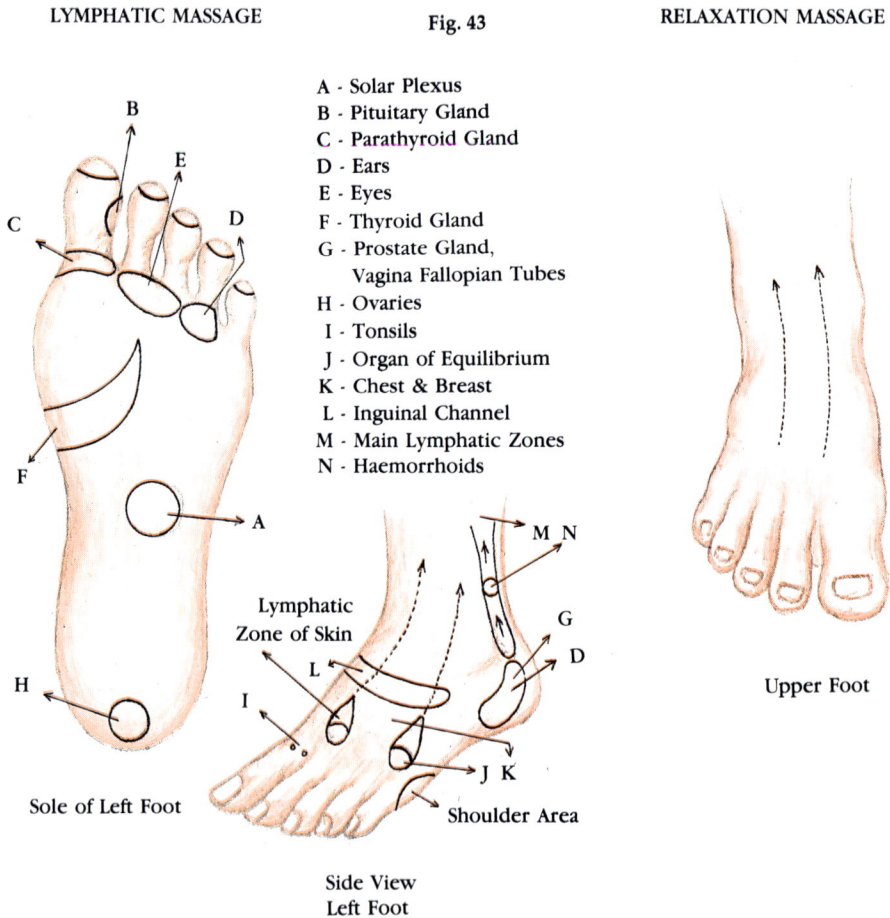

LYMPHATIC MASSAGE   **Fig. 43**   RELAXATION MASSAGE

A - Solar Plexus
B - Pituitary Gland
C - Parathyroid Gland
D - Ears
E - Eyes
F - Thyroid Gland
G - Prostate Gland,
     Vagina Fallopian Tubes
H - Ovaries
 I - Tonsils
 J - Organ of Equilibrium
K - Chest & Breast
 L - Inguinal Channel
M - Main Lymphatic Zones
N - Haemorrhoids

Lymphatic
Zone of Skin

Upper Foot

Sole of Left Foot

Shoulder Area

Side View
Left Foot

Relaxation massage. During relaxation one often visualizes images and wonderful colors. Massage very lightly and gently with soft circular movements along the main lymphatic lines on the upper side of the feet towards the ankle (see Figure 43). Always begin simultaneously on the outer area of both the feet, then toward the big toe in the direction of the ankle. Finish with a gentle stroke along the top of both the feet beyond the feet. Massage for 10 minutes.

This massage is effective for autogenous training or meditative practice as it enhances one's entry into a quiet calmness. Before rising, hold the sole of the patient's foot with one hand, making a fist with the other hand and rolling it along the sole from the toes to the heel.

Procedure

The therapist needs to do certain exercises to strengthen fingers and palms.

1. Holding both palms (inner side) against each other, press against one another with considerable pressure.

2. In a similar exercise, hold the fingers including the thumbs against each other and exert similar pressure.

3. Holding the fingers of one hand with the other bend them backwards. Do the same with the other hand.

While exerting pressure on the selected pressure points, certain factors are important such as the patient's age, physical condition, kind of ailment, duration of the ailment, situation of the point, and so on. In case the patient is being treated for the first time or if the patient has acute pain or swelling exists at that point, the underlying muscles are weak or even when the corresponding system or organs are heavily damaged due to the ailment, then the patient should be given light pressure. The pressure may be more or hard if the patient is not too tired, the state of the disease is chronic, or if the patient has no other complications. The average duration for giving pressure is between 6 to 7 seconds each time. The process can be repeated 3 to 4 times.

The therapist/masseur/masseuse should bear in mind certain important instructions before giving the treatment.

1. Treatment should not be given under high stress or strain conditions.

2. Acupressure should not be taken on a full stomach (wait for 2 hours after a meal) nor on an empty stomach.

3. In case of any medication, wait for 2 hours before treatment.

4. After a hot water bath, wait for half an hour before treatment.

5. Under normal circumstances, acupressure should not be given to pregnant women.

6. Do not use acupressure if an injury or a fractured limb is located in the exact same spot.

7. Do not treat sciatica or serious injury to any of the vertebrae.

As mentioned in other forms of treatment, the expulsion of waste or toxic matter from the body during the treatment can take place in many forms. Be alert to the signs and symptoms of expulsion of waste products.

Like Shiatsu, these acupressure therapies are specialized. The information given here is only the tip of the iceberg. For your reference and ready reckoning see Figures 36, 39 and 40 showing both acupressure as well as reflexology points.

APPENDIX B

YOGA NIDRA

After spiritual energy massage the patient should rest for about 15 minutes during which he can practice yoga nidra. In short, yoga nidra is that state which is between sleep and Samadhi, a state of equilibrium. When a person sleeps, he or she is there but is not conscious. In yoga nidra the person is in a half-sleep and half-waking state. It is a state wherein a person can be resting completely with very little sleep and yet remain fully aware and conscious of the surroundings. This patient benefits from the point of view that along with complete rest and good sleep, he/she experiences a high state of consciousness.

The practice of yoga nidra is beneficial because in that state a person may be able to have access to solutions, answers, ideas, plans, and so on which may not be available in the waking state. During this conscious sleep the patient/client can enjoy a keen state of awareness while the whole body, mind, and nervous system get complete rest. In this state, all events, incidents, and happenings are recorded by the subconscious by getting back into that state of yoga nidra. By practicing this technique one will realize that 10 minutes of yoga nidra is far superior to three hours of ordinary sleep. Several techniques can help you practice yoga nidra. Without going into too much detail, here are some very simple tips.

The best time to practice yoga nidra is early in the morning. After ablution, sit down and meditate for about half an hour in the calm and quiet atmosphere of the morning. Meditate at a fixed hour everyday. Spread a clean carpet or mat on a wooden cot or on the floor. Block the ears with cotton balls to keep all sounds out and then close your eyes. If necessary, use a soft pillow under the head.

With eyes closed, concentrate on the eyebrow center, which is the ajna or the inner eye chakra. In the wakeful state, the mind functions mainly focusing on this chakra. The ancient yoga books say that while dreaming, the mind is focused on the vishuddhi (throat) chakra. During deep sleep the mind goes to the anahata (heart) chakra. Breathe diaphragmatically and take three deep breaths, breathing in and out slowly. Concentrate entirely on the breath. Do not let thoughts disturb you. After a few moments, gradually move your concentration to the throat or vishuddhi chakra. Visualize the moon at the vishuddhi, continue breathing diaphragmatically and take three deep breaths. Shift your concentration to the anahata chakra. The breathing should be deep and continuous.

An important point to note is that this exercise is bound to induce sleep but the patient must overcome sleep in order to continue with yoga nidra. Also make sure to breathe in and out in a deep rhythmic fashion. Breathe, concentrating on every part of the body, from the top of the head to the tips of the toes. Carry your concentration via the breath, first through the left side of the body and then through the right side. You will realize that you have attained a very alert state of mind when you return to the ajna chakra. This alert state of the mind is the opposite of the heart beat which is very soft and slow indicating that the heart is at almost complete rest. After exactly 10 minutes, you will wake up. If you do not wake up it means that you are sleeping and not in yoga nidra.

When you wake up, gradually, bring your attention to the reality around you, and do it systematically. Be aware of your body, the external sounds, both inside and outside the room and slowly get up. As you get up, with your eyes closed, rub the entire length of your body including the face and head, with the palms of your hands. Practicing yoga nidra daily at a fixed time is extremely beneficial.

KAYAKALPA

In my opinion, authentic Kayakalpa is not practiced anywhere today. I am explaining the process briefly for your information. Kayakalpa is the science of rejuvenation. The *Charaka Samhita* says that the rishis (sages of yore) returned to their original abodes in the mountains, after having lived an urban life for a considerable amount of time. The Himalayas offered them solace and comfort, especially after the hectic, erratic, and luxurious urban life, whose evils weaned them away from Mother Nature. The calm, serene, rejuvenating atmosphere of the mountains and their wilderness lured them back to a quiet life.

One of the original elixirs of life, soma, which is a creeper, came from these regions in the Himalayas. A principal nostrum of a branch of Ayurvedic medicine which used soma came to be known as kayakalpa (the science of rejuvenation). Somarasa, which belongs to rasayana (the science of potency) is made from sovereign herbs that grow in the Himalayas. These include asparagus, yam, and many others. Rasayana, which in Sanskrit means rejuvenation or "the path of juice", is a process whereby one can replenish the quality and quantity of the body's fluids. The process of aging causes the body to lose its juices and fluids and, therefore, wither. With the help of rasayana, one can retain, regain, or enhance one's youth, strength, stamina and virility.

Kayakalpa is a combination of two words, kaya meaning body and kalpa meaning rejuvenation or the medical treatment of the sick. The *Sushruta Samhita* says that the gods created soma to prevent the death and decay of the body. For the practice of kayakalpa, a special structure is constructed which has an inner chamber surrounded by seven walls. This is built at a site protected from all climatic conditions and external influences. It is provided with all the required accessories. Attendants and helpers should be acquired before the patient is administered the somarasa. Then at an auspicious hour, on an auspicious day, marked by favorable astral combinations and calculations, the person desirous of undergoing the treatment should enter the innermost chamber. The person is admitted only after having cleansed the system thoroughly with purgatives and having adhered to proper diet restrictions. At this stage, the juice is extracted from the soma plant with a golden needle in a gold vessel. This juice is then given to the patient.

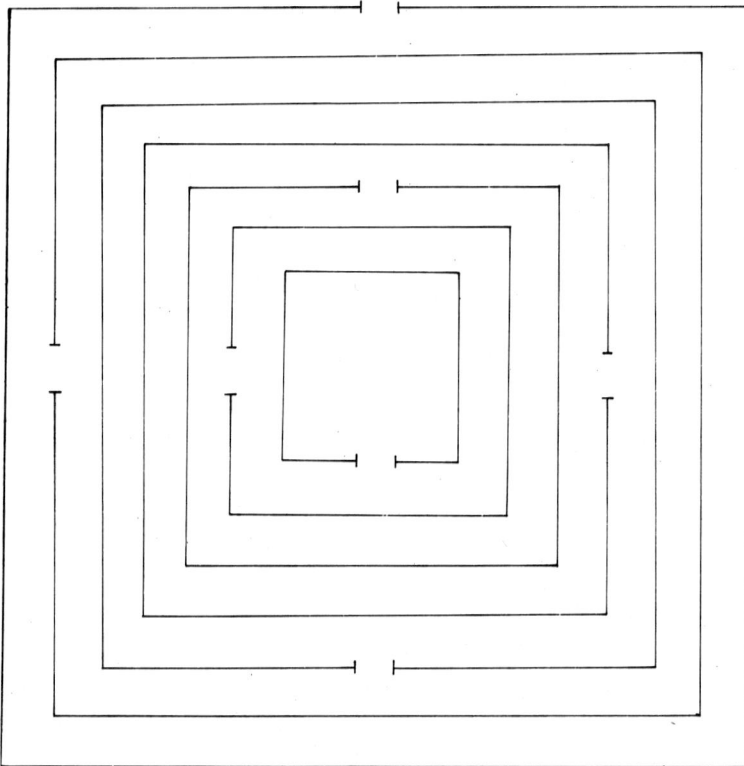

ROOM FOR KAYAKALPA

The patient is expected to be in the innermost chamber for the next eight days, during which the person has to observe paramount duties of truth, non-violence, detachment to possessions, and celibacy, along with minor duties such as cleanliness, happiness, austerity, self-study, and thoughts of God. The diet consists mainly of milk, which is boiled and cooled and is given only at specific times.

When the patient digests the somarasa, he undergoes a spate of vomiting. This continues for about seven days and all the impurities that have been accumulated over the years are expelled from the body. This elimination takes place in the form of worms, blood, mucus, loose stools etc. In this manner the whole body is thoroughly cleansed.

At the end of seven days, the patient loses weight and becomes completely withered. The skin looks chapped and cracked and the teeth, nails and hair begin to fall off, though the vital spark is retained by the potency of the somarasa. On the eighth day, the patient is bathed in milk and covered with sandal paste. From then on the muscles of the body begin to show signs of fresh and vigorous growth. New teeth will be formed, symmetrical, hard, and strong, as clear as diamonds. This happens around the 17th or the 18th day. Fixed, glossy, and coral colored nails begin to grow and so will the hair. New skin will assume the soft hue of a lotus.

The patient is then moved into the second chamber for the next ten days. The diet is gradually changed, though it is still regulated. The patient should not, however, contemplate himself in the mirror and should follow the duties mentioned earlier.

After the entire treatment, the patient is allowed to resume normal life very gradually. The patient can now enjoy a new and youthful body. Such a person is protected against the negative aspects of fire, water, poison, weapons, and so on. The person will also develop great muscular energy. The presence of such a person gladdens the heart. It is believed that the entire knowledge of the vedas and their allied branches instinctively dawns on such a person. The *Sushruta Samhita* also says that the soma plant is invisible to the impious, ungrateful and spiteful individuals.

CHARTS OF MARMAS

This table shows you the 107 marmas, in the three main classifications, at a glance.

Regional	No.	Structural	No.	Prognosis	No.
Upper and Lower limbs	44	Muscular	11	Slow death	33
Abdomen	3	Ligamental	27	Disability	44
Thorax	9	Joints	20	Pain	8
Back of the trunk	14	Blood Vessels	41	Vishalyaghna Marma	3
Head and Neck	37	Bones	8	Sudden death	9
Total	107		107		107

The following table is in the prognostic format and is according to the corresponding element of nature. The kinds of effects have been divided into five groups.

No.	Name of Marma	Element	Prognosis
1	Asadhya Pranahar Marma (Sudden death)	Fire	Just as fire diminishes quickly, injury by fire can lead to sudden death
2	Kalantara Pranahar Marma (Slow death)	Fire and lunar, which is watery	Immediate death will not occur. But due to the loss caused by fire and the gradual loss of water, death occurs
3	Vishalyaghna Marma (Death on removing the weapon)	Air	Removing any foreign body from a wound causes the air to escape and the contact with the marma is lost, thus causing death

| 4 | Vaikalykar Marma (Disability) | Water | Maintains life by the virtue of water which is relatively stable and has cooling qualities. It causes disability. |
| 5 | Rujakar Marma (Pain) | Fire and Air | Causes only pain |

I have divided the 107 marmas in the regional format with the appropriate figures, so that it becomes easy for the masseur to locate the required marma. In the normal condition all the areas of marmas can be massaged without more pressure.

UPPER AND LOWER LIMBS (Figure 6)

No.	Name of Marma	Place	No. of Marmas	Regional	Structural	Prognosis
1	Talahrat 1/2 angula*	Both palms	2	Middle of the palm straight below the middle finger	Muscular flesh	Slow death, death if timely treatment is not given
2	Talahrat 1/2 angula	Both soles	2	Middle of the sole straight to the middle toe	Muscular flesh	Slow death, death if timely treatment is not given
3	Kshipra 1/2 angula	Both hands	2	Between the thumb and the index finger	Tendon	Death if timely treatment is not given. Regular massage gives relief.

4	Kshipra 1/2 angula	Both legs	2	Between the big toe and first toe	Tendon	Slow death
5	Kurcha 4 angula	Both hands	2	2" above Kshipra	Tendon	Disability —regular massage gives relief
6	Kurcha 4 angula	Both legs	2	2" above Kshipra	Tendon	Disability —regular massage gives relief
7	Kurchesin Kurcha Kakyam 1 angula	Both hands	2	At the end of the palm near the wrist	Tendon	Pain
8	Kurchesin Kurcha Kakyam 1 angula	Both legs	2	At the end of the sole near the ankle	Tendon	Pain
9	Mani Bandha 2 angula	Both hands	2	On the wrist joints	Joint	Pain
10	Gulpha 2 angula	Both legs	2	On the ankle joint	Joint	Pain
11	Indra vasti 1/2 angula	Fore-arm	2	Middle of the forearm	Muscular flesh	Slow death —timely treatment may give relief
12	Indra vasti 1/2 angula	Fore-leg	2	Middle of the fore-leg	Muscular flesh	Slow death —timely treatment may give relief

13	Kurpara 3 angula	Arm	2	On the joint of the elbow	Joint	Disability
14	Janu	Leg	2	On the joint of the knee	Joint	Disability
15	Ani 1/2 angula	Arm	2	3" above Kurpara	Tendon	Disability
16	Ani 1/2 angula	Leg	2	3" above Janu	Tendon	Disability
17	Urvi 1 angula	Upper arm	2	In the middle of the upper arm	Blood vessels	Disability
18	Urvi 1 angula	Thigh	2	In the middle of the thigh	Blood vessels	Disability
19	Lohita 1/2 angula	Armpit	2	In the armpit	Blood vessels	Disability
20	Lohita 1/2 angula	Knee socket	2	In the thigh socket	Blood vessels	Disability
21	Kaksha-dhruk 1 angula	Above the armpit	2	Above the armpit	Ligamental	Disability
22	Vitapa 1 angula	In the middle of both legs	2	Between the scrotum and hernia	Ligamental	Disability

*Angula is a measurement from the tip of the thumb to the tip of the thumb's joint.

ABDOMEN

No.	Name	Place	No.	Regional	Structural	Prognosis
1	Guda (anus) 4 angula	Anus	1	Around the anus	Muscular flesh	Death
2	Vasti (pelvis) 4 angula	Waist	1	In the middle of the waist	Tendon	Death
3	Nabhi (navel) 4 angula	Middle of the torso	1	Between the upper part of the belly, navel and the abdomen	Ligamental	Death

THORAX

No.	Name	Place	No.	Regional	Structural	Prognosis
1	Hriday (heart) 4 angula	Dia-phragm	1	In the middle of the thorax where the stomach and the chest join	Blood vessels	Death
2	Sthana mula (root of the breast) 2 angula	Breast	2	2" below each breast	Blood vessels	Slow death

3	Sthana rohita 1/2 angula	Breast	2	2" above each breast	Muscular flesh	Slow death
4	Apastamba 1/2 angula	Breast	2	In the middle of each breast and collar bone	Blood vessels	Slow death
5	Apalapa 1/2 angula	Chest	2	On both sides of the middle bone of the chest	Blood vessels	Slow death

BACK OF THE TRUNK (Figure 7)

No.	Name	Place	No.	Regional	Structural	Prognosis
1	Katika taruna 1/2 angula	Back	2	On both sides of the spine near the hips (loins)	Bone	Slow death
2	Kukun- dara 1/2 angula	Back	2	On both sides of the spine above the loins	Joint	Loss of feeling

3	Nitamba 1/2 angula	Back	2	On both sides of the abdomen above the loins	Bone	Slow death
4	Parswa sandhi 1/2 angula	Back	2	At the root of the parsukha bone, 2" above Nitamba	Blood vessels	Slow death
5	Brihat 1/2 angula	Back	2	Between each breast and the spine	Blood vessels	Slow death
6	Amsa phlaka 1/2 angula	Back	2	On both sides of the spine and trikasthi above the tail bone	Bone	Disability
7	Amsa 1/2 angula	Back	2	Below the head behind the neck near each shoulder	Ligamental	Disability

NECK

No.	Name	Place	No.	Regional	Structural	Prognosis
1	Manya 4 angula	Neck	2	On both sides of the tubular vessels of the throat, on the outer vessels of the jaw	Blood vessels	Loss of speech
2	Neela 4 angula	Neck	2	Near the Manya marma on the inner side of the jaw	Blood vessels	Loss of speech
3	Matruka 4 angula	Neck	8	On both sides of the tubular vessels of the throat on the 4 vessels of the tongue and nose	Blood vessels	Sudden death
4	Krikatika 1/2 angula	Neck	2	On both sides of the joint of the head and neck	Joint	Disability

HEAD (Figure 8)

No.	Name	Place	No.	Regional	Structural	Prognosis
1	Vidhura 1/2 angula	Head	2	Below both ears	Tendon	Loss of hearing
2	Phana 1/2 angula	Head	2	On both nostrils near both the eyes	Blood vessels	Loss of the sense of smell
3	Apanga 1/2 angula	Head	2	A little below the eyebrow center	Blood vessels	Loss of sight
4	Avarta 1/2 angula	Head	2	A little above the eyebrow center	Joint	Loss of sight
5	Sankha	Head	2	Between each ear and the end of the eyebrow (temple)	Bone	Sudden death
6	Utkshepa 1/2 angula	Head	2	Above Sankha marma near the hairline	Ligament	Vishal-yaghna marma
7	Sthapani 1/2 angula	Head	1	Between both the eyes, at the root of the nose	Blood vessels	Vishal-yaghna marma

8	Shringa-taka 4 angula	Head	4	The place where vessels of the tongue, eyes, ears and nostrils meet	Blood vessels	Sudden death
9	Seemanta	Head	5	On the head	Joint	Slow death
10	Adhipati 1/2 angula	Head	1	In the head	Joint	Sudden death

NAMES AND ADDRESSES OF AYURVEDIC MEDICAL CENTERS IN KERALA

1. VAIDYARATNAM P.S. VARIER'S ARYA VAIDYASALA,
   KOTTAKKAL P. O. KOTTAKKAL
   District : MALAPPURAM, KERALA STATE (INDIA)
   Phones: 04934-2210, 2216, 2219, 2561-2564 & 2571-2573

   (EPABX-TDBX) 200 lines

   Branches with Phone Nos:

KOZHIKODE	0495/75666 & 63664
PALGHAT	0491/23104 & 27084
TIRUR	04938/2231
ERNAKULAM	0484/352674 & 360026
TRIVANDRUM	0471/78439
ALWAYE	04854/3549
MADRAS	044/6411226
KANNUR (CANNANORE)	0497/64164
COIMBATORE	0422/24724
NEW DELHI	011/4621790

2. WARRIER AYURVEDA KENDRAM,
   XXV/1105 PAZHAYANADAKKAVU,
   TRICHUR 680001 (KERALA, INDIA)
   Phones: 0487/27462
   Branches:
   EDAPAL 04939-523
   KOZHIKODE 0495-62293
   ERNAKULAM 0484-362225

3. ARYA VAIDYA PHARMACY (CBE) LTD.
   P.B. NO. 3769, 1382 TRICHY ROAD
   COIMBATORE - 641018
   Phone: 216006
   Nursing Home: ARYA VAIDYA CHIKITSALAYAM &
   RESEARCH INSTITUTE
   P.B. NO. 7102 COIMBATORE-641045
   Phones: 213188 & 214953

Branches:
BOMBAY 22 SION WEST Phone: 4078187
BOMBAY 14 SECTOR 9 CBD, NEW BOMBAY
NEW DELHI 5 B-A WEA KAROL BAGH
Phones: 5745296, 5785687

4. SREE SANKARA AYURVEDA VAIDYASALA
    PERUNNA CHANGANACHERY - 686102
    KOTTAYAM, KERALA (INDIA)
    Phones: 04824-21154/20954

Though it is a small Ayurvedic Center-cum-Nursing Home with 15 beds, all kinds of Ayurvedic medicines required for treatment are prepared there. The work on a project for holistic treatment including music therapy, yoga and meditation is being started on the top of a beautiful mountain which is very attractive to the foreigners.

Shirovasti (Vasti for the head). Shirovasti is most important of all external uses of oil and is a rather serious treatment which gives relief from all diseases of vata in the head, headache, vata oriented cataract, earache, humming of the ears, deafness, spasm of the jaw-bones, haemiplegia (turning the face to one side due to paralysis), dryness of the mouth or nose, numbness of the head and all ailments based on the cranial nerves.

The patient is cleansed with Snehana (oleation) and Swedana (sudation) on an auspicious day. After noon the patient is seated on a stool facing west in the room chanting some prayers. When the patient sits ready on a stool, fold the cloth in 2 inches broad and tie it round the head above ears. The cap, made of stiff, smooth cowhide both ends open, is to be slid down the head over the cloth tied around the head, properly fitted. An unguent pad is wrapped around it, neither loose nor too tight. Apply the black gram paste at the lower end of the cap so that the oil poured on the head does not trickle down. The agreeably warmed up oil be poured slowly over the head after ensuring the head held straight. The level of the oil should be about 2 inches (5 cm) above the crown. The remaining oil may be kept on slow fire to keep the same warm continuously. When the oil over the head cools off remove it by soaking it up with the piece of cloth and replace it with the remaining same warm oil. This process is continued till the end. Generally in excess vata the duration is about 50 minutes, in excess pitta is 40 minutes and in excess kapha is 30 minutes. And for a healthy patient 5 minutes is enough. The other indication is, when the kapha loosens and starts draining out through the nose and mouth, it is to be stopped. Then the oil is removed quickly with the cloth, the cap and band untied and removed. The head must be swabbed clean and the neck, shoulders, ears, face and back of the neck are to be massaged for some time. The patient be smeared with oil again and bathed. If bath is prohibited (taboo) the patient must be rubbed down with a clean towel without further inunction, to remove the oil completely and he should lie down and relax completely. This treatment can continue 3, 5 or 7 days according to the nature of the disease, but never more than 7 days. Diet and other restrictions are also to be observed. If the treatment is done properly the benefit is as follows:

"The oil in the crown overcomes the falling, greying and other discolouration and cracking of the hair and all vata ailments of the head. It also bestows liveliness to the organs, a clear voice and firm jaws and strength of the head."

Infertility Problems

In 1994 a lady medical doctor from Goa, after reading my book, "Techniques of Massage" wrote a letter congratulating me. She asked me whether there is any solution for women's infertility problems. Generally I suggest to consult any Ayurvedic doctor for solution.

In U.S.A., a lady asked me about her infertility. I gave her some suggestions which the couple followed strictly and after a year she gave birth to a baby. Thanking me she sent a greeting card. The suggestions are:

1. Abstain from sex for two weeks, it is a must.

2. Reflexology:

(a) The couple should stimulate the genital reflexes every morning and night 5 minutes on each foreleg inside the edge of the bone and the muscles between the strip of knee and the ankle bone 7 points on equidistance.

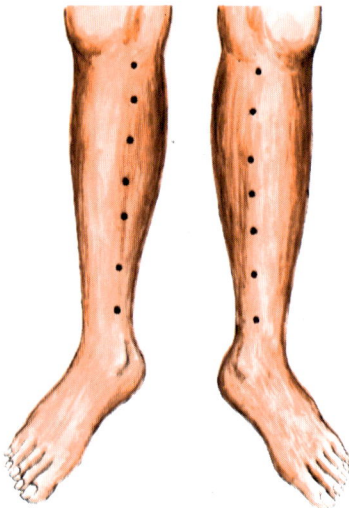

7 points on equidistance between the knee and the ankle bone on the side of the big toe between the bone and muscle

Fig. 44

(b) Pumping should be done 15 times on each of the points of spine reflexes, adrenal gland, solar plexes, colon and pancreas and also all the points of the big toes. The points of genital reflexes, kidney, urinary bladder, uterus, vagina, prostate penis, and pancreas are on both the legs (see Fig. 46). Pumping should be done 15 times on each of these points. Always at the end do tapotement and effleurage for a minute or two. Finish with a joint affirmation "we are going to have a beautiful child." It must also be affirmed upon arising and retiring.

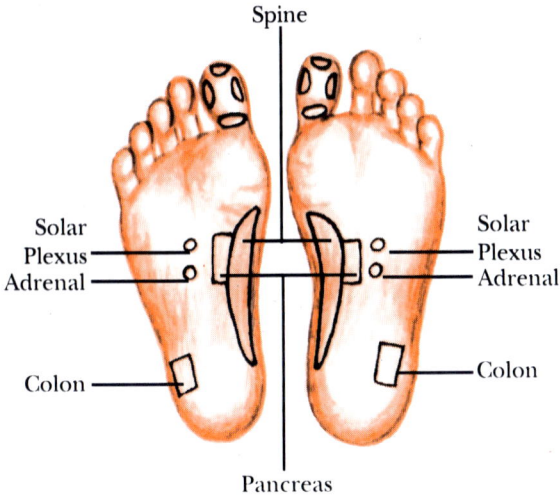

Spine

Solar
Plexus
Adrenal

Colon

Pancreas

Fig. 45

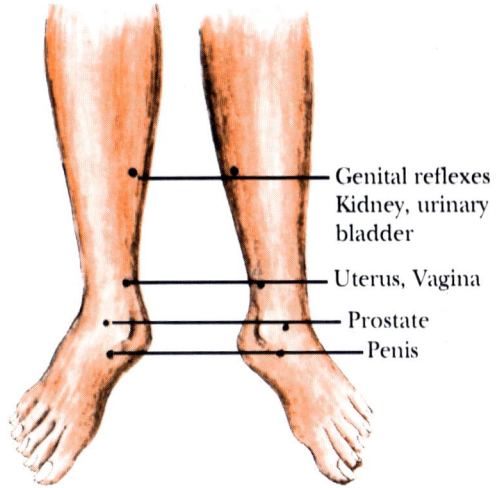

Solar
Plexus
Adrenal

Colon

Genital reflexes
Kidney, urinary
bladder

Uterus, Vagina

Prostate
Penis

Fig. 46

3. Diet: Eat a menu high in raw foods such as whole grains, nuts, cabbage, fruits, leafy greens, onion and garlic.

Daily eat at least 1 tablespoon sunflower seed, sesame and pumpkin seed each.

4. Daily take a balanced dose of vitamin E and B complex, and M2-Tone an Ayurvedic drug prepared from several Indian herbs by Charak Pharmaceuticals.

5. Fast a day before resuming sex activities.

6. First massage each other's feet focussing on the points prescribed above and end with firm affirmation at night before resuming sex activities.

7. Each should feel the energy going down from the top of your head into your heart and reproductive organ.

8. Continue this regimen until you have success. Have fun and have a baby.

Exercise to Strengthen Reproductive Organs

(a) *Individually (each)*

1. Stand up placing your hands on your knees. Take a deep breath and exhale fully.

2. On exhalation lean over and squeeze up your productive organ and anus as tightly as possible through holding back a bowel movement.

3. Fully release the muscles. Squeezing and releasing of these muscles and organs stimulate the blood flow, nutrition and tone. Repeat 25 times.

4. Inhale as you stand up, relax and do a healing visualization. Imagine the inner environment of your productive organs and observe them functioning normally.

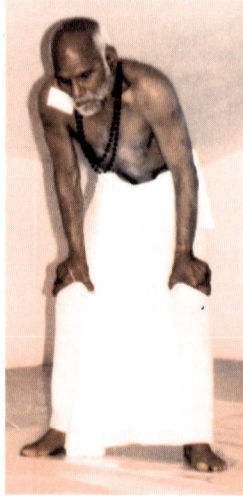

Photo 47

(b) *Jointly*

5. Both of you sit face to face on a mat on the floor stretching the legs forward so that each other's soles of the feet touch together. Then bend forward and hold each other's hands together. Gently lift up both of your feet together and keep mutual eyes-contact, while breathing deeply together for 1 to 3 minutes. This exercise mutually stimulates each other's foot reflexio and creates a bond of shared energy.

Curing Infertility = M2-Tone

Infertility is mainly a result of hormonal imbalance, emotional trauma or malnu-

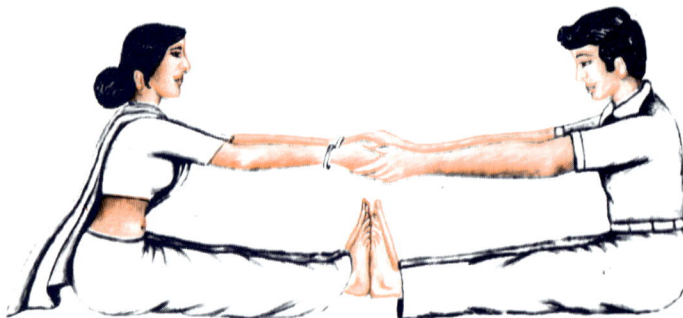

Fig. 47

trition. Such problems associated with menstruation and infertility are comprehensive and holistic. M2-Tone tablet or syrup (an Indian herbal drug manufactured by Charak Pharmaceuticals) provides this.

Irregular menstruation is cause of concern for most of the women. At times patients complain of dysmenorrhoea. These conditions are associated with emotional disturbances like anxiety, depression, insomnia, lethargy and fatigue which further aggravate this delicate feminine balance. Even emotional disturbances can precipitate these menstrual problems. The female body obtains the necessary body-building blocks through nutrition. Deficiency of vitamin B12 or Folic Acid also causes anaemia. A common problem occurring in women anaemia will result in short supply of oxygen and hence energy. It can slow down the function including the hypothalamus and pituitary.

M2-Tone is a non-hormonal, non-steroidal, ayurvedic medical preparation. By giving this to female the rate of conception becomes better. It also improves the endometrical receptivity, regulates menstrual cycles, corrects oxygenic insufficiency, relieves emotional stress, encourages optimal endometrical proliferation, normalises the quality of menstrual flow, corrects ovarian insufficiency, creates a fertile intra-uterine environment conducive to conception and full-term gestation, improves the chances of conception, inhibits excessive uterine contractions and provides relief from painful abdominal cramps.

Treatment for Male Impotence

1. Treat the cervical region by pressing and massaging.

2. Lie prone (i.e. face downwards) position. Treat the medulla oblongata region and dorsal, lumbar and sacral regions. Do this 3 minutes. Then press the points of the back (see Fig. 48).

3. Lie on spine position (face up).

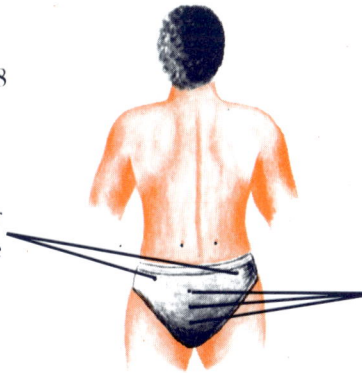

Fig. 48

The points on the upper part of each buttock are namikoshi points.

3 bone knots of the vertebra after the coccyx are the sacral region. The points on both sides of the 5th bone knot after coccyx are the lumbar region points.

Press (pump) the pubic bone that relates to puberty 3 minutes and also press

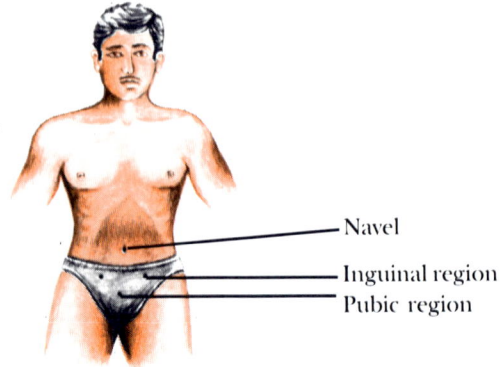

Fig. 49

Navel

Inguinal region
Pubic region

(pump) the inguinal points shown in Fig. 49 another 3 minutes.

Treatment for Agnesia (Inability to Fertility)

Agnesia is seen sometimes 50% in a male and 50% in a female. The same treatment is given to females as suggested to males.

1. Treat cervical region and medulla oblongata.

2. Let the patient lie down on a prone (face downwards) position. Then press (pump) the points of dorsal region, vertebra, colon, lumbar region, iliac crest, sacral region, gluteal region and namikoshi region as shown in Fig. 50.

3. Let the patient lie down on spine (face up) position. This treatment is only for women.

Female back   Female front

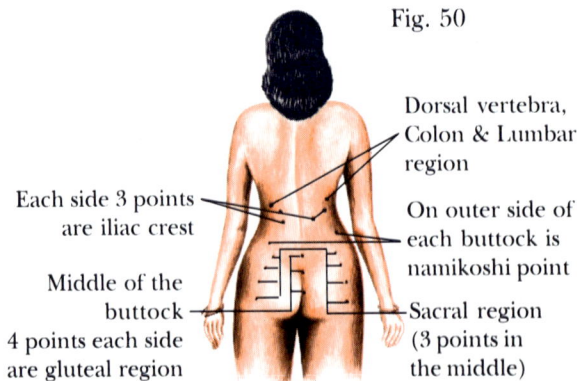

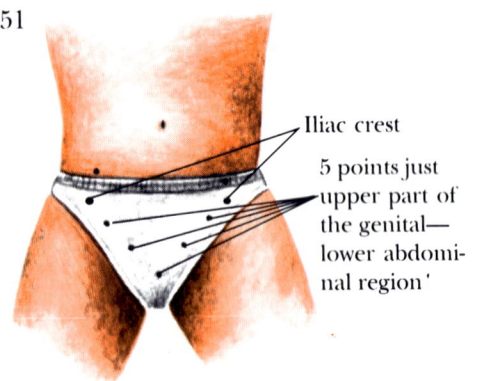

Fig. 50   Fig. 51

Dorsal vertebra,
Colon & Lumbar
region

On outer side of
each buttock is
namikoshi point

Each side 3 points
are iliac crest

Middle of the
buttock
4 points each side
are gluteal region

Sacral region
(3 points in
the middle)

Iliac crest

5 points just
upper part of
the genital—
lower abdomi-
nal region'

So-ham—Sah = He; Aham = I

Why don't I know myself who am an embodiment of Existence-Knowledge-Bliss; the words Existence, Knowledge and Bliss denote an individual Entity. What is consciousness is Bliss and the witness is illuminating all things like sun. Everything is known through the light of consciousness which is the self.

Give up the misconception identifying the self with the body, the senses, the mind, the intellect and the vital force and always night and day, by renewing everything that may stand in the way of constant meditation, know yourself to be Existence-Knowledge-Bliss the witness of the intellect.

The gross body is not the self as it is possessed of form etc., and also because it is a modification of the ether and other great elements.

Thus ascertain for the discrimination of the self from the subtle body, that I the seer of the senses am not the senses themselves and know for certain that I am neither the mind, nor the intellect, nor the vital force.

Convince that I am also not the combination of the gross and the subtle bodies and ascertain accurately by means of inference that I the seer am quite distinct from the seen.

Know yours to be one owing to whose proximity alone non-conscious entities like the body and the senses are able to function by way of acceptance and rejection.

Have the firm conviction that I am one with the changeless innermost self that moves the intellect like the magnet (loadstone) moving the iron.

It is really the consciousness of the self that makes the body, the mind etc. appear to be conscious like the fire making a red-hot piece of iron look like fire.

I am not other than the consciousness which is the self illumining the modification of the mind such as my mind went elsewhere but it is now brought to rest.

It is due only to the consciousness of the self that intellect and its functions are known.

I am the changeless self that is immediately cognized and that illumines the 3 states of waking, dream and sleep as well as the appearance and disappearance of the intellect and its modifications.

The self, an embodiment of consciousness is the illuminator of the gross and the subtle bodies and therefore quite distinct from it just like a lamp lightening a jar which is known to be different from it.

I am the seer the object of supreme love with regard to which there is the earnest desire I may be always.

Consciousness which is of the nature of a witness is what is meant by I. Witnessing again is nothing but knowingness on the part of the self as one devoid of all changes.

I am quite different from the body, the senses, the mind, the vital force, the ego and is absolutely free from the six changes: birth, phenomenal existence, growth, passing from one state to another, declension and destruction to which all non-conscious things are subject.

The all-pervading being absolutely free from all the impurities, transmigratory existence, having the qualities of not being seen, even free from the taint of darkness, having no greater bliss than itself, the embodiment of Existence, Knowledge and Bliss for its peculiar definition to be the universal self.

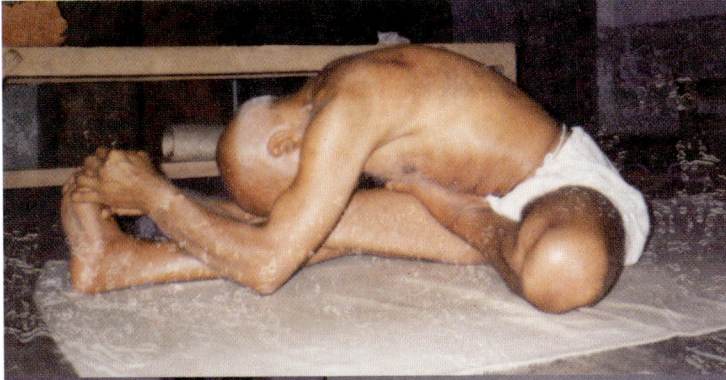

48

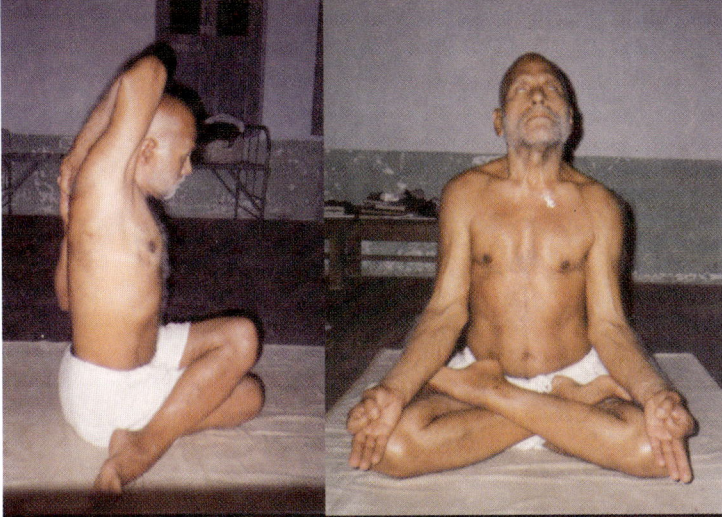

49

54

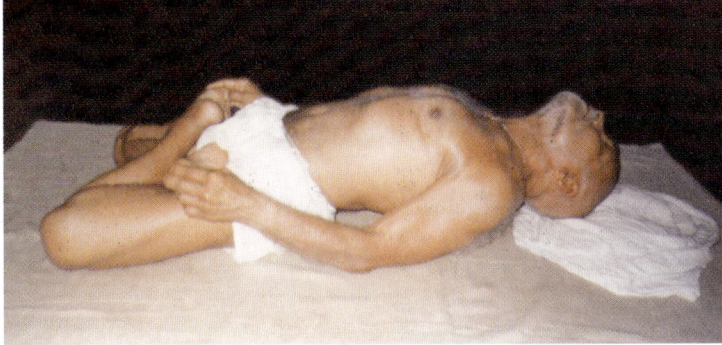

53

48. Janushirsasana (See page 112 Col.8)

49. Gomukhasana (See page 112 Col.8)

53. Mayurasana (Matsya Mudra) (See page 112 Col.8)

54. Sadhana (See page 112 Col.8)

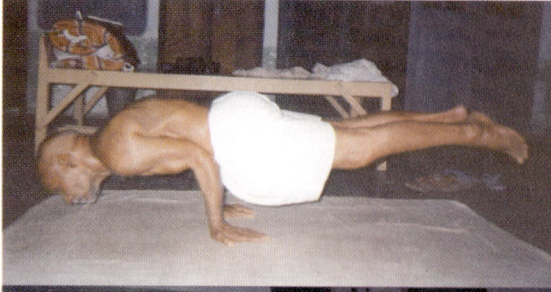

50

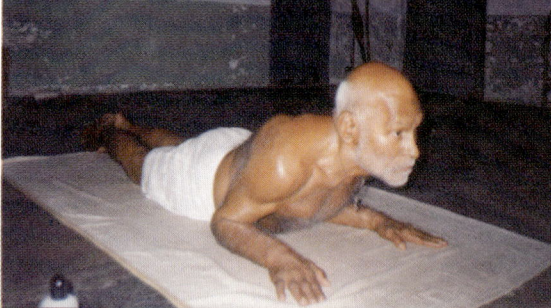

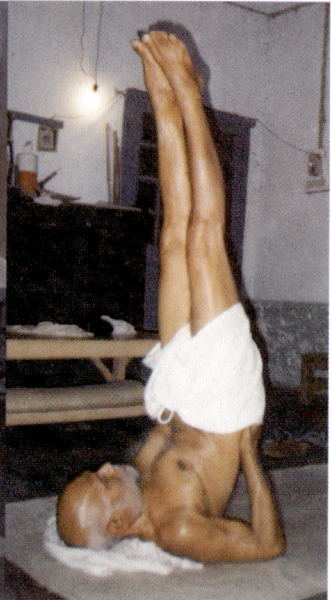

51

52

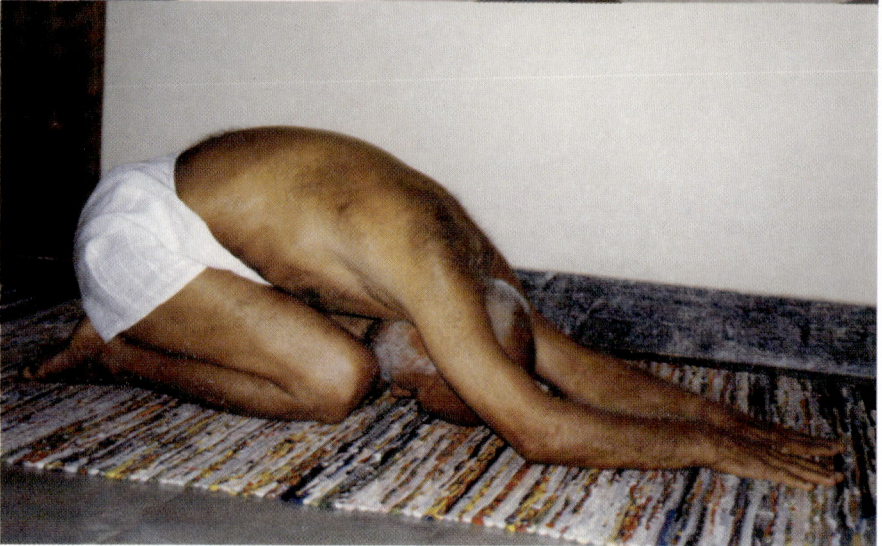

55

50. Mayurasana (See page 112 Col.8)

51. Bhujangasana (See page 112 Col.8)

52. Sarvangasana (See page 112 Col.8)

55. Shashankasana (See page 112 Col.8)

BIBLIOGRAPHY

I	Arya Vaidya Sala Kottakkal	i) Anatomical and Physical Significance of Marma ii) Chikitsa Samgraham (Malayalam) (Physical Medicine and Rehabilitation) iii) Tridosha Theory iv) Arya Vaidyan Quarterly Magazine
II	J.W. Amstrong	The Water of Life — a Treatise on Urine Therapy
III	Swami Shankaradevananda Saraswati & Swami Satyananda Saraswati, Bihar School of Yoga, Mungher	Amaroli
IV	D.R. Dhiren Gala & Sanjay Gala Gala Publication	Health in Your Hand
V	Bhagavandash Lalitesh Kashyap	Basic Principles of Ayurveda
VI	Swami Rama — The Himalayan International Institute of Yoga Science and Philosophy of the U.S.A. Honeysdale Pennsylvania	Path of Fire and Light Vol. 1 & 2
VII	Marianne Uhl — Lotus Light Publication, Wilmont U.S.A.	Chakra Energy Massage
VIII	Lucinda Liddel with Sara Thomas, Gaia Books Ltd., 9th Edition, 1990	The Book of Massage
IX	Harish Johari — Munshiram Manoharlal Publications Pvt. Ltd., New Delhi	Ancient Indian Massage
X	Wataru Ohashi	Do it Yourself SHIATSU
XI	Sarva Seva Sangh Publication, Varanasi	Vaijnanik Malish (Hindi)

INDEX

Acupressure   121-126
   abdominal ailments   125-126
   general treatment   124-125
   nervous disorders   126
Almond oil   72
Amritadi tailam   75
Anu tailam   76
Asana Eladi tailam   72, 73
Asana Manjishthadi tailam   73
Asana Vilwadi tailam   72
Auto massage   66-67
Ayurveda
   ancient history   29-30
   diagnosis   33-34
   Tridoshas
      kapha   31-35
      pitta   31-35
      vata   31-35
Ayurvedic herbs   96
Ayurvedic massage
   auto massage   66-67
   Ayurvedic oils   72-76
   beauty massage for women and men
      60, 65-66
   benefits of   36, 83-84
   cold massage   60
   color and their effects   77-79
   doing massage with legs   88
   general guidelines
      for children   42
      for masseur/masseuse   36-42
      for the patient   42
      for women   42
   general oils   71-72
   guidelines for massage of different
      parts of the body   44-60

massage movements   67-71
   effleurage   67
   friction wringing   68
   kneading   68
   petrissage   67-68
   tapotement   69-71
   massages of Kerala   85-88
   solar energy oils   76
   ubatans (pastes)   79-80
   urine therapy massage   80-83
Ayurvedic oils   72-76
   for fractures, dislocation and swell-
      ing   74
   for head massage   72-73
   for mental illness   75
   for paralysis, polio, rheumatic pains
      and acute gout   74-75
   for retaining youth   76
   for skin diseases   73-74

Bala tailam   75
Baladhatryadi tailam   73
Balaguluchyadi tailam   73
Balaswagandhadi tailam   73, 75
Bhringamalakadi tailam   73
Brahmi tailam   73
Butter   72

Chakras   104-108
   Ajna Chakra   107-108
   Anahata Chakra   107
   Bindu Visarga Chakra   108
   Manipura Chakra   106-107
   Mooladhara Chakra   105-106
   Sahasrara Chakra   108
   Swadhisthana Chakra   106
   Vishuddhi Chakra   107
Chandanadi tailam   73, 75
Coconut oil (*Doorvadi*)   71, 73
Charaka   30

Cold massage 60
Color therapy 77-79
Coriander oil 72

Dhanwantharam tailam 74
Dhara 86-88
Digestion
 six factors for 35

Effleurage 67
Endocrine glands
 adrenal & pancreas glands 110
 gonads 110
 pineal gland 110
 pituitary gland 110
 prostate gland 110
 thymus gland 110
 thyroid gland 110

Food combinations
 dos and don'ts 98-102
Foods
 effects of different types of
  foods on human
  constitution 96-98
Friction wringing (*Marshanam*) 68

Gandha tailam 74
Gandhaka tailam 73
Ghee 72
Guidelines for massage of
 abdomen 47-48
 arms 46
 back 53-54
 chest 48
 feet 44
 head, neck and face 54-60
 knees 45
 lower legs 44
 upper legs 44
 waist 48, 53

Healing through massage
 Ayurvedic herbs 96
 case study summaries 89-90
 diseases of the abdomen
  constipation 93

obesity 94
piles 94
prostate 94
sleeplessness 94
slimness 94
diseases of the nerves
 arthritis 91
 high blood pressure 92
 leprosy 92
 madness 92
 nervous tension 92
 paralysis 91-92
 polio 91
 rheumatic pain 91
 rheumatism 91
 sciatica 90-91
food combinations 98-102
general injuries
 compound fracture 95
 fractures 95
 inflammation 95
general rules
 lower body 90
 upper body 90
Human physiology 17-23
 bones 20
 circulation 20-21
 heart 21
 joints 20
 lymphatic system 21
 muscles 20
 nervous system 21-22
 skin 22-23

Jatyadi tailam 74
Jivantyadi tailam 75
Jivantyadi Yamakam 75

Kachoradi tailam 75
Karpasasthyadi tailam 74
Kayakalpa 85, 134-136
Kerala
 Ayurvedic massages of 85-88
Kneading (*Mardanam*) 68
Kshara tailam 73
Ksheeraba tailam 74

Kumkumadi tailam 76
Kundalini 103-104

Lemon juice 71
Linseed oil 71

Mahabala tailam 75
Mahamasha tailam 75
Maha Narayana tailam 74
Malatyadi tailam 76
Marmas, science of 23-28
    blood vessel marma 27
    bone marma 27
    joint marma 27
    ligament/tendon marma 27
    muscle marma 26
    prognostic marmas 26
    regional marmas 23
    structural marmas 23
    vishalyaghna marma 26-27
Massage, history of 13-17
Mustard oil 71

Narayana tailam 74
Nasarsas tailam 76
Navarakkizhi 86
Nilibhringadi tailam 75
Nimbadi tailam 73

Olive oil 72

Petrissage (*Peedanam*) 67-68
Pinda tailam 74
Pizhichil 85
Prabhanjana vimardana tailam 74
Pumpkin seed oil 72

Rasnadi tailam 75
Reflexology 126-132
    guidelines for massage 129-131
    massage instructions 129
    procedure 131-132

Sahacharadi tailam 75
Saubhagyavardhana tailam 76
Sesame oil 72

Solar energy oils 76
Spiritual energy massage
    Chakras 104-108
        Ajna 107-108
        Anahata 107
        Bindu Visarga 108
        Manipura 106-107
        Mooladhara 105-106
        Sahasrara 108
        Swadhisthana 106
        Vishuddhi 107
    Chakras and endocrine glands 109-112
    Kundalini 103-104
    techniques of 112-120
Sushruta 30

Tapotement 69-71
Taste
    six types of 35
Tekaraja tailam 75
Tridoshas
    kapha 31-35
        five types of 34-35
    pitta 31-35
        five types of 34
    vata 31-35
        five types of 34
Triphaladi tailam 73
Tungadrumadi tailam 75

Ubatans (pastes), use of
    for beauty 80
    for general purposes 79
    for pimples and boils 80
    for rheumatism 79
    for skin 79
Urine therapy massage 80-83

Vatamardana tailam 75
Vilwapatradi tailam 73
Vinobaji 67

Yoga nidra 133-134
Yuvatyadi tailam 76